Contents

Parents talking

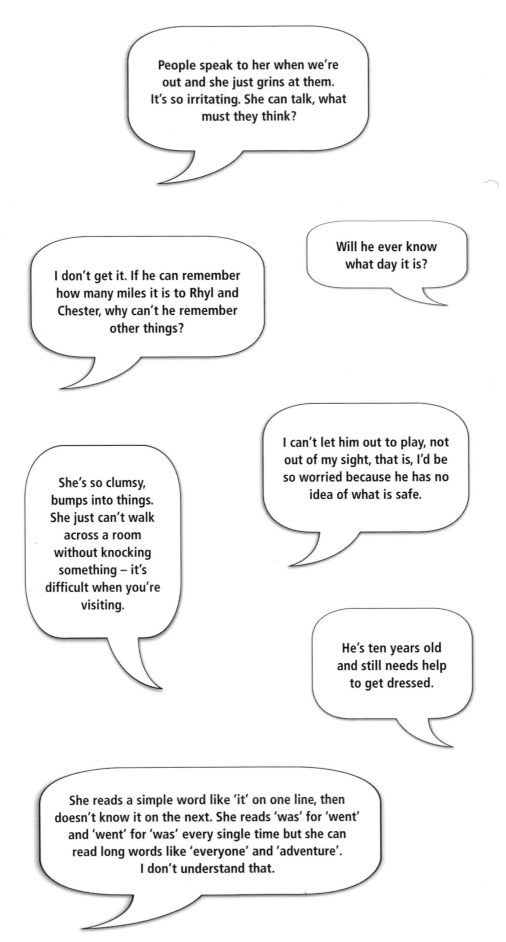

People speak to her when we're out and she just grins at them. It's so irritating. She can talk, what must they think?

I don't get it. If he can remember how many miles it is to Rhyl and Chester, why can't he remember other things?

Will he ever know what day it is?

She's so clumsy, bumps into things. She just can't walk across a room without knocking something – it's difficult when you're visiting.

I can't let him out to play, not out of my sight, that is, I'd be so worried because he has no idea of what is safe.

He's ten years old and still needs help to get dressed.

She reads a simple word like 'it' on one line, then doesn't know it on the next. She reads 'was' for 'went' and 'went' for 'was' every single time but she can read long words like 'everyone' and 'adventure'. I don't understand that.

Supporting Children with Speech and Language Impairment and Associated Difficulties

Jill McMinn

Suggestions for supporting the development of language, listening, behaviour and motor skills

The *Questions Publishing Company* Ltd

Birmingham

2002

The Questions Publishing Company Ltd
Leonard House, 321 Bradford Street, Digbeth, Birmingham B5 6ET

First published in 2002

ISBN: 1-84190-083-4

Editorial team: Amanda Greenley
                       Linda Evans

Design team: James Davies
                       Iqbal Aslam
                       John Minett

Cover photograph by: Stuart Mills

With thanks to staff and children at Acton Park Infant School.

Printed in the UK

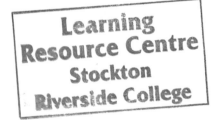

I wouldn't mind but we've done colours, colouring, jigsaws, songs, everything since she was a baby and she still says our red car is blue.

She talks rubbish, it doesn't make sense but she just carries on, she doesn't realise we're not following. Then she gets in a temper after when we don't do what she wants.

He has no friends – he's desperate to have friends.

He's been shown where to put his tongue and how to put his mouth, so why can't he do it?

We've always had them, animals I mean, and she's always helped with them but she can't tell you a cat is an animal.

She interrupts all the time, doesn't wait her turn. It's so embarrassing.

She looks fine, just like her sister, so what's wrong? Why does she have to go to another school in a taxi?

His baby cousin understands us. But he just looks blank.

Acknowledgements

Thank you to all the parents who have shared their experiences with me; their worries when things were difficult and their joy when things went well. You have given me a valuable perspective and taught me a lot. The time spent in teaching your children with speech and language difficulties has been extremely enjoyable and rewarding.

I owe a great deal to all those colleagues in education and health who have supported me in developing various ideas. Particular thanks go to Jane Williams, who has encouraged me to develop inclusive, whole-school systems of support, and Angela Hughes, who is always ready with wise words of constraint for my wilder ideas!

Last of all, thank you Kate, for your encouragement and support, notably with many cups of excellent tea and thank you David, for your patient and talented advice on my word processing.

Introduction

By the time children start school at the age of four or five, most of them are fairly well organised. They have sorted, classified and categorised information into the right places in their minds. They can use language to communicate and socialise. They can use language to learn.

'P.E. worns out me.'

This book is about a different group of children; children who are disorganised, but quite overcome by disorder. Children who can't make sense of the world. They are totally distracted by all the information presented to them, so much so that they can appear not to be paying attention or even to be deaf. In fact, they are often paying too much attention to one word or phrase, trying to make sense of it, while the rest of the sentence goes unheeded.

'My dad went hammer and hammer bang went wood down.'

These are children who are lost in space and time. They can't recall the sequence of things, don't know what day, season or year it is, and are confused by *today, yesterday* and *tomorrow*. They muddle *up* with *down, behind* with *in front, right* with *left*. They can't visualise their own space or their own body moving in space. They misplace their belongings. They are clumsy, losing their balance. They may not be able to co-ordinate several things at once. Their timing is always off.

'I feel look not book reading now.'

These are the children who know what they want to say but whose language comes out muddled or unintelligible.

'On Saturday next tomorrow I will went.'

They talk about 'aminals', 'hopsitals' and 'spickets'. They say *'Mrs Minn I've shifin'* instead of *'Mrs McMinn I've finished'*.

They have a lot to say but it is impossible to decipher what they are telling us.

'Mrs Minn I've shifin.'

They can quickly complete tasks and want to describe what they have done, but it is very difficult to follow their description and consequently they cannot easily demonstrate knowledge and understanding.

'Tom nursery has gone.'

They know what it is to feel wet yet call wet things 'dry', they call breakfast 'dinner' and horses, 'cows'.

They won't accept broken biscuits because a biscuit is supposed to be round, and they may freeze when faced with a choice of two things – unable to select one.

'Him not got a throwinger.'

They get bound up in the detail rather than seeing the whole.

Language is central to learning and to life in general. It helps to shape the daily routines of health and welfare, as well as social relationships in the family, at school and at work.

'Language is so tightly woven into human experience that it is scarcely possible to imagine life without it.'
Steven Pinker (1994)

This book offers information, guidance and examples of good practice to teachers, learning assistants and parents working with children who have speech and language difficulties. With appropriate help, these children can be taught to make their speech clearer, improve listening and co-ordination skills and to make more sense of their world. When they are given opportunities to develop and show their knowledge, children with speech and language impairment can and do learn.

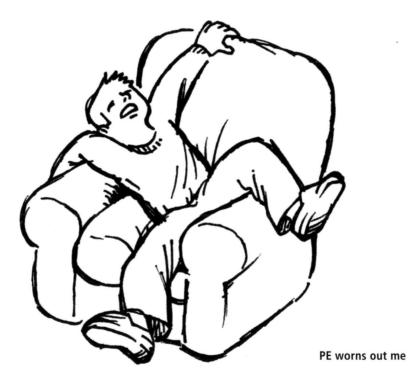

PE worns out me

'Language is not solely a means of communication, it's also a powerful cognitive tool, serving as a means of mental representation, hence influencing thinking and memory'

Morag Donaldson (1995)

What is Speech and Language Impairment?

Joy Stackhouse describes Speech and Language Impairment (SLI) as:

'A developmental disorder characterised by the late appearance and/or slow development of comprehension and/or expression in a population of children who are otherwise cognitively, emotionally and physically intact'
(Acton Speech and Language Conference, July 1997)

This impairment may be called 'severe' because its effects are widespread, impeding communication and learning. It may be called 'specific' because it may not be linked to any other major difficulty. However, the term can encompass a wide range of difficulties, some of which also stand on their own and some of which are also associated with other conditions and areas of special educational need. (See diagram over the page.)

Not all pupils with speech and language impairment will attend a specialist class; a significant number will be in mainstream classes. Many Key Stage 1 teachers believe that they have steadily increasing numbers of pupils with some degree of speech and language impairment, certainly with poor listening skills. This may be so, or we may be getting better at recognising these difficulties. Depending on how it is defined, estimates of the prevalence of speech and language impairment vary between 3% and 15%.

So we are talking about a wide range of problems experienced by a significant number of children. Some of these children will be considered as speech and language impaired, others will be experiencing more general difficulties with learning, and some will have speech and language difficulties as part of other identified impairments such as hearing loss. Some of these children may spend a short or a longer time in specialist classes, others will be in mainstream classes for most, if not all of their education. It is important therefore, to raise awareness of these difficulties and provide some ideas of how best to support children in mainstream schools.

Children with speech and language impairment (SLI) are a challenging yet stimulating group to work with. To be successful in teaching them you need enthusiasm, patience, flexibility and a large bank of ideas. The resources we have collected and developed may therefore be useful to mainstream and to specialist colleagues who work with children who need support in a range of areas:

The NHS Centre for Reviews and Dissemination suggests that 6% of children will have some kind speech, language or communication difficulty at some stage in their life. David Hall (1996) suggests that 1 in every 500 children will have a severe long-term difficulty.

The number of potential cases of children with speech and language impairment is high. A conservative estimate suggests 1-2% but well designed studies suggest 7% may have some kind of speech and language impairment.

(Law, J. (ed) 2000)

- Expressive Language:
  Speech, Vocabulary, Grammar

- Receptive Language:
  Listening, Following instructions, Memory

- Social Use of Language:
  Behaviour

- Developmental Co-ordination Difficulties

Speech and language impairment can encompass a wide range of difficulties

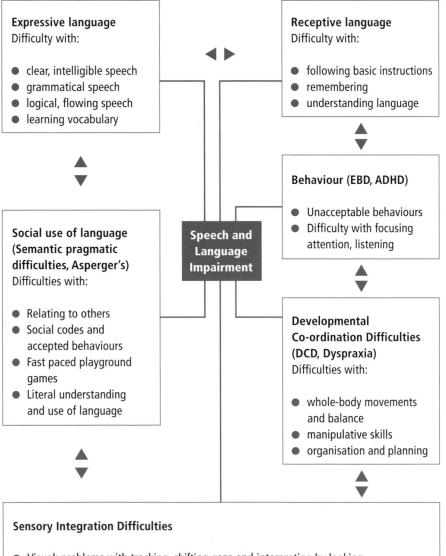

Expressive language
Difficulty with:

- clear, intelligible speech
- grammatical speech
- logical, flowing speech
- learning vocabulary

Receptive language
Difficulty with:

- following basic instructions
- remembering
- understanding language

**Social use of language
(Semantic pragmatic
difficulties, Asperger's)**
Difficulties with:

- Relating to others
- Social codes and
  accepted behaviours
- Fast paced playground
  games
- Literal understanding
  and use of language

**Speech and
Language
Impairment**

Behaviour (EBD, ADHD)

- Unacceptable behaviours
- Difficulty with focusing
  attention, listening

**Developmental
Co-ordination Difficulties
(DCD, Dyspraxia)**
Difficulties with:

- whole-body movements
  and balance
- manipulative skills
- organisation and planning

Sensory Integration Difficulties

- Visual: problems with tracking, shifting gaze and interpreting by looking
- Auditory: problems with locating sounds, identifying and discriminating between sounds
- Taste and smell: over or under-reaction to particular tastes and smells, leading to
  restricted diet and dislike of 'hands-on' activities
- Tactile: over or under-reaction to touch, dislike of hair or nails being cut, lack of
  awareness of nose running or food spilled on clothes, fiddling with everything
- Vestibular/proprioceptive difficulties with balance and body awareness

Expressive Language

Speech production, vocabulary and grammar

Children with expressive language difficulties may be very difficult to understand.

They may:

- use speech that is unclear or garbled
- talk too loudly or too softly, too quickly or too slowly, hardly at all or not at all
- use very few words and lots of gestures
- miss out words or invent words
- muddle or misuse syllables within words and words within sentences
- muddle pronouns, tenses and questions
- have trouble recalling certain words, saying nothing or using a word that sounds nearly the same or one that means nearly the same
- lack the understanding of conversational rules and, though eager to have a conversation, make little sense whatsoever
- be unable to make links and connections with language and therefore be unable to explain or describe clearly
- give unexpected answers, since they may interpret words literally
- lack understanding of social rules and codes.

In a busy classroom, children who have just one or two of these difficulties may be overlooked. They may give yes and no answers when questioned directly and may talk infrequently but be considered as merely shy or reserved. Children with more severe difficulties are easier to identify.

Whether experiencing minor or severe difficulties, such children will need direct support to acquire and use language.

Speech production

The children with speech production difficulties are fairly easy to identify because they are difficult to understand and may even be totally unintelligible. Sometimes, family members may learn to understand their own child in context, but such children probably still remain unintelligible to other people, including their teachers. If they cannot make themselves understood it is very difficult for them to learn alongside their peers in a mainstream class. They may have associated difficulties with the structure of language and they may go on to have literacy difficulties, more commonly called Specific Learning Difficulties (SpLD) or Dyslexia.

These children need a very specific programme of therapy to enable them to learn how to articulate speech sounds. Single speech sounds

'ga go gan?'
(Can I go in the sand?)

'Mrs McMinn the water bowl is stuck and it's a flood.'
(Mrs McMinn, the sink is blocked and there's a flood.)

2

must be explicitly taught, followed by blended sounds as they occur in different positions in words. Speech and language therapists often teach pairs of sounds (c/g, t/d, p/b) that are made in the same place in the mouth but one is softer, less stressed than the other. They may talk about *loud* and *soft* sounds, and *long* and *short* sounds. They will usually practise sounds in isolation (/p/ then with open vowels pee/pay/poh/pie...) then with another consonant at the end (peed/paid/pohd/pied) and so on. They will encourage good posture and breathing throughout.

This sounds straightforward but it is extremely hard work. Most children need to go over and over aspects of this work before it begins to be automatic. They do not automatically know how to shape their mouths or where to place their tongues, and often they have to slow right down in their speech production while they do these things. The children have to take some responsibility for their own improvement and want to make their speech clearer. This is a mature concept for very young children.

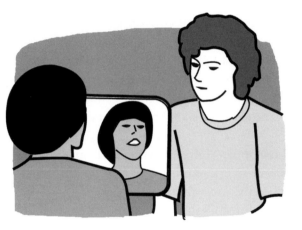

When a child is working on articulating particular speech sounds it helps to work with the speech and language therapist (SALT). Within a specialist language class the therapist and the teaching staff will plan and work together. In mainstream settings, it would be immensely helpful if a key worker in school could work with the child for a short time each day; this could be the SENCo, class teacher, NNEB or teacher's assistant. The therapist will have very limited time available for each child and will probably ask parents to help as well. She will usually set out a detailed programme for the child and it is clearly of most benefit if daily practice is possible. (It is useful to know the order of acquisition of sounds for speech so you can follow the SALT programme with more understanding and also to see what stage your pupil(s) have reached. See Appendix 1.)

'Me not play her, her rough.' (I'm not playing with her, she's rough.)

Practice

It takes a lot of practice and encouragement for a child to carry over what has been introduced in a therapy session into free speech. If you are aware of the programme and, for instance, know that a child has been practising an initial /c/ sound, then every time 'Can I...' is used you can be ready to encourage the use of this sound. Similarly, when reading with the child, you can expect, encourage and praise the use of target sounds.

In addition, look for times in the course of regular school activities when you can practise the target sounds in ordinary talk. This sometimes means employing techniques more often used with much younger children, such as prompting, re-stating and expanding what the child has said in a supportive way. Try to praise good attempts, rather than concentrating on correcting errors, and help the child to feel relaxed and happy enough to repeat target sounds in regularly used phrases in class. Sometimes it is appropriate to link speech work with alphabet, spelling and reading tasks in class. Be ready to do this but discuss it with the therapist first.

Be prepared for the times when you will not understand what the child is saying and be ready to acknowledge this and to re-assure the child. It is pointless to pretend to understand, as the child will know you don't. Better to be ready to say:

- 'Can you show me?'
- 'Can you draw it for me?'
- 'Children, can you help? See if you know what John is saying.'

Sometimes other children are really good at interpreting because they are on the same wavelength. (Of course the child needs to feel relaxed and the class needs to be geared up to supporting him, it has to be done in a friendly, supportive way.)

- Whatever the outcome, praise the child for having a try, but if you have not understood, say something like, '*I'm sorry I couldn't understand. You are working really hard to make your talking clear and it is getting clearer all the time*'.
- Then try and have a talking time with a shared and familiar context as soon as possible e.g. do some art work together, read together or play a game together so you can have a successful conversation. Of course this will not be possible every time but it has to happen enough to motivate the child to become intelligible.
- Give extra encouragement to pupils with speech difficulties with regard to their reading. As you tune in to their speech you will be able to assess if they are reading the words accurately. Start with a core sight vocabulary, as you probably do anyway, before using 'sounding out'.
  (See first key words, Appendix 2)
- Consider using a phonic/alphabet system that uses visual clues such

'Ta, ti to too toiti?'
(Can I go to the toilet?)

as Jolly Phonics. Accept a best effort from your pupil with speech difficulties. This is where you need to liaise with the SALT, but also enable the child to show what he knows through using pictures or letters.

If a child stutters there are some ways you can help.

- Don't focus on the stuttering or label the child as a 'stutterer'.
- Don't ask him to slow down or think about what he is saying.
- Do give him time and attention, with the same chance to talk as everyone else in the group. Listen to what he says and answer or comment on the content, not on how it was said.
- Do notice which situations seem to worry him the most and consider how to overcome these.

Your speech and language therapist can give more detailed advice. Children who stutter can be lacking in confidence, and very vulnerable, isolated and subject to name-calling and 'put-downs'. (A useful and informative resource is produced by the British Stammering Association.)

Generally, in the area of speech production, you can help by including some rhythm work in your music lessons. How we speak – the expression and inflection we use – is linked to our sense of rhythm. Many children with speech and language difficulties have a very poorly developed sense of rhythm. Tapping out different rhythms and a steady beat to different songs or music, and playing softly and loudly, or fast and slow, can be fun and helpful. Rhythm and rhyme go well together so you could also choose some words or rhymes that include particular speech sounds that a pupil is working on and say and tap these. This also gives a chance for some positive affirmation to your pupil about his speech work. (Some rhymes are given in Appendix 3)

Rhythm games
- Clapping round circle. First child claps once, then next child and so on, like a ripple. This requires good looking and focused attention and aims to develop group identity, and the group working together. If the children get good at this, make it harder by using two or more claps or a clapped rhythm.
- Tap children's names, topic or curriculum vocabulary or phrases from songs. Have these written and the rhythm marked in some way, dots or musical notes.
  Say and clap the rhythm of the words three times, whisper and clap, then think and clap.
  Or say and clap hands, say and clap knees, say and clap thighs, say and clap the floor. Then repeat this pattern but say and clap hands, then think and clap knees, thighs, floor.
- Leader claps a rhythm and children echo it back.
  When they are confident at this introduce '*Don't do this*'. Have a card with the words '*Don't do this*' and the rhythm shown in some way, dots or musical notes. Now if the children hear this rhythm they don't echo it.

- Play tap, tap say – start a rhythm, tapping knees twice then stretching hands forward in front to mark a pause. When the children have got this rhythm then introduce saying a word in the pause, taking it in turns round the circle. These can be on a given category – vehicles, food, colours – whatever you wish to work on. The aim is for no duplication, although at first it may be necessary to accept some duplications. It is useful to practise by counting round the circle or saying own names to get the feel of it first.
- Use a large dice, throw it then clap the number.
- Use well-known rhymes and songs to emphasise rhythm. Pound fists or clap hands together on stressed words.

'I wan go girs gu egun moogi.'
(I want to go first but everyone's moving.)

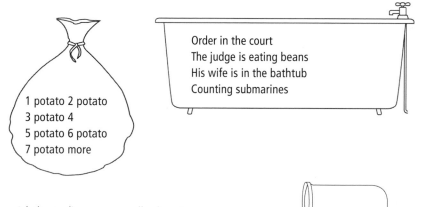

1 potato 2 potato
3 potato 4
5 potato 6 potato
7 potato more

Order in the court
The judge is eating beans
His wife is in the bathtub
Counting submarines

A baby sardine saw a small submarine
And was scared and looked through a peephole
Oh come, come, come said the sardine's mum
It's only a tin full of people

The King or Queen's rhythm

Have a crown to pass around: each child in turn is the king or queen and chooses an action. (At first have these ready – bowing, clapping, waving, curtsying, marching, saluting, then the children can add some more.) All do the action in time/in the rhythm of the word – bowing, bowing, bowing or saluting, saluting, saluting.

- Sing and use tuned instruments for pitch work to help develop the high and low tones of talk, the music of talk (prosody).
- Include some tapping out of syllables in your music or literacy sessions, this helps with spelling as well. Tap the children's names. Multi-syllabic words can be tapped out too; these can be curriculum vocabulary which helps with this learning too. Use picture references and, at first, mark the number of syllables.

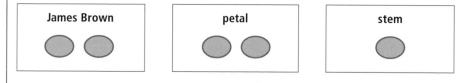

| James Brown | petal | stem |

- Learn some rhymes/poems connected with curriculum areas that include particular sounds (Appendix 3).

Vocabulary

Some children need support to acquire and use even common vocabulary and language concepts, and many older pupils still need concrete experiences to grasp new vocabulary.

Use a full multi-sensory approach wherever possible and consider the levels and ways of learning, when planning how to help children learn and understand vocabulary. Use real or replica items wherever possible, so the children can handle them, look at them, hear them, talk about them in as many ways as possible. When this is not possible, photos or clear pictures are the next best. Follow-up writing and reading tasks can be structured to include specific vocabulary.

- Consider the key vocabulary that your pupils need to know in each subject area (See Appendix 2). Be realistic about what they will be able to learn or they may well 'switch off' and learn very little or nothing at all.
- Teach vocabulary words before presenting them in lessons. As part of this, teach them how to answer questions (Appendix 4). When the children are answering or asking questions, give them 'think about' prompts:

  What category does it belong to?
  What is it made from?
  What does it go with (brush with hair/teeth/dustpan)?
  Where could it be seen?
  Who made it/uses it?
  What does it sound/smell/feel/look like?
  Is it the **name** of something, **describing** something or about **doing** something (noun/adjective/verb)?
  What sound does it start/end with, what does it rhyme with, how many syllables has it got?

- Plan short but frequent practice times for this vocabulary. For instance, sing or chant the days of the week, the months of the year and the countries of Great Britain regularly during register/ carpet time.
- Discuss familiar words when they are presented in new contexts, (light = not dark, light = not heavy).
- Instead of allowing free choice writing, ask for a piece about things that are rough and smooth, hot and cold, old and young, etc.
- Many concepts can be explored during science activities – wet/ dry, hard/soft, rough/smooth etc.
- Consider a particular vocabulary list to work on with each class topic, and let parents know what it is so you can work on it together. If they are made aware of it, parents can help at home by mentioning and practising target vocabulary in everyday situations.
- Have a word or words of the week.
- Practise using imagery and 'thinking' pictures. Tell a short story, then show the children a picture or a set of pictures that illustrate

'My mum took me.'
'Mmm, took you where?'
'Yes.'
'Where did you go?'
'Yes, I went and it was so good.'

this, then hide the picture(s) and tell the story again asking them to think the pictures. As they become more confident ask them to think their own pictures and tell the group about these. They can be encouraged to 'think pictures' whilst reading or tackling comprehension tasks.

'He's very sizes.'
(He's very tall.)

- Older children may find it helpful to draw up charts of key vocabulary, which can be added to and then used for reference. They could use a vocabulary reference book with their own terms and alongside them, a choice of alternatives e.g. sadness (sorrow, despair, gloom); happy (joyful, cheerful, ecstatic)

- **Vocabulary.** Older pupils need to explore additional vocabulary through use of antonyms, synonyms, root words, categorisations, associations and multiple meanings.

- Use commercial games and adapt others to learn and extend vocabulary. **Descriptive games** can be played with a range of pictures carefully selected to meet current language targets. There are commercial sets available, but newspapers, comics or wrapping paper are rich sources.

- **4 Facts.** Have four counters and a set of model animals or pile of animal pictures in the middle. Each child in turn takes an animal and names it, then tries to give four facts/sentences about it. As they do so, put down a counter for each fact. When they have given four facts ask the rest of the group what else they know about the animal.

- **Verb game.** Have verbs written out on cards and practise performing these. After enough practice one pupil can perform a verb for the others to guess. It may be necessary to have a selection of the verbs on display at first so that the players can guess from a given selection, rather than from memory. An adverb game can be played in the same way.

'Struggles, look,
struggles.'
(Squirrels, look,
squirrels.')

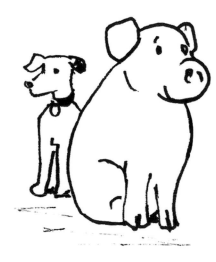

- **Guess the animal.** Have a set of animals hidden from general group view. Each child in turn comes out to choose an animal, keeping it hidden. Either have the child describe the animal for the others to guess or have the children ask questions to work out what the animal is. This game can be used for any vocabulary.

- **Word Association.** Take a class word such as 'family' and collect as many words as possible for that family – baby, mum, dad, brother, aunt…

- **Word Association 2.** Take a word, perhaps from the current topic, and using prompts, find as many other associated words as possible e.g. wood

  Family/category – plants or growing things

  Function/what does it do, what do we do, who does this – provides home for animals, looks good, gives us wood to make things

  Place or time – wood, garden, forest…

  Appearance/parts, look, sound, smell, texture, size, shape – trunk, branches, leaves or rough bark, green leaves…

  Reaction/how do you feel about it…

- **Pairs.** Have pairs of cards with one on view or one of each in a pile from which the children select in turn and have to give the pair.

  Table and… Cup and… Postman and…

- **Twenty Questions.** Play this first with the items to be guessed in full view. As the children become more confident it can be tried with the items hidden or just thought of.

  Start at an easy level – 'I'm thinking of something grey with four legs' – and progress to – 'I'm thinking of something, it's animal' – and twenty questions are allowed in which to guess it. This helps develop questioning skills and can also be linked to current topic work. The definitions of the four possible categories of animal, vegetable, mineral and abstract would need to be discussed first. Older pupils may enjoy a simplified/customised version of Taboo or may be able to play the game itself.

- **Oral games.** Differentiation of work needs to include consideration of difficulties with literal interpretations, double meanings, colloquialisms, embedded clauses and other complex structures. Use or adapt oral games to target these. Try including one or two common expressions or sayings in each bank of topic work or linked to what you say in class e.g. 'soft as butter/hard as nails' or 'pull your socks up'. These can be discussed, demonstrated and illustrated. (A useful booklet called *Figures of speech* is available from AFASIC. We have also found these useful: *'A Bird in the Hand'* by Nigel Snell published by Hamish Hamilton 1986 ISBN 0 241 11815 8 and *'Quick as a Cricket'* by Audrey Wood published by Child's Play 1982 ISBN 0 85953 306 9)

'Ben toilet gone.'
(Ben has gone to the toilet.)

Grammar

There are various elements of grammar that cause problems for some children. Most of these need direct attention and would be included in the therapist's programme but also need to be included in class work.

Positional prepositions

(In, on, under, behind, in front, next to, across, against, far, near etc.)

Some children need a lot of practice at these.

- They can be targeted directly in PE warm-up sessions, Maths activities or Geography activities when pupils can move behind, in front, over or under, or position apparatus.
- For younger children it is helpful to have a bag of items and containers to manipulate, puppets can be used too. The children can be directed to *'put the dog in the car'*, etc.
- Older children need to be exploring the wider and less obvious meanings of these positional words e.g. **in** a box, **in** the garden, **in** a fix, **in** a muddle, **in** a mood etc.

Personal pronouns

Many children with speech and language difficulties muddle these. 'Me' is used when it should be 'I'; Mr, Mrs, Aunt and Uncle etc. will cause problems as well as she/he and her/him etc. They can be practised in context at home and school and pointed out in reading, writing and speaking activities.

- Each child can carry out an action, or mime an occupation for the others to guess using he/she.
- A commentary on a video or description of a picture can be given using target pronouns.
- Photographs of a child's extended family or a fictitious family can be used to target family words like aunt/uncle, cousin, brother/sister.
- Multiple mime: this is one of our made-up games where the group mimes a chosen job or action in a range of ways with appropriate individual and group commentary. So one girl mimes and says, '**I** am cooking', then the group chorus '**she** is cooking'. One boy mimes for **I** am cooking/**he** is cooking. Several children for **we** are cooking/ **they** are cooking and everyone for **we** are cooking. We have added **my** meal is delicious/**our** meal is delicious/**their** meal is delicious and included associated phrases to practise **his/her/mine/ours**. It is helpful to have picture reference clues in sight at first. We have adapted this to practise adjectives, adverbs, position words and a range of targeted vocabulary in conjunction with pronouns. In this way we can re-visit areas of language again and again, which is just what our children need. Older pupils could play it as a guessing game.
- Change the words of well-known songs to practise he/she or other

'I wented to the swimming.'

'You went to the swimming pool, and what did you do there?'

'I am swimming now and she is splashing me but I do not like that.'

personal pronouns e.g:

'Megan put the kettle on, **she** will put the kettle on, **she** will put the kettle on, **we'll** all have tea.

James take it off again, **he** will take it off again, **he** will take it off again, **we'll** all go away.'

● **His/hers** or **him/her** can be practised with a set of objects, each child chooses one and places it in front of themselves. Go round the circle chanting 'The blue pencil is **his**', 'The red pencil is **hers**', about the items.

Or 'The blue pencil is by **him**', 'the red pencil is by **her**'. Or, Teacher: 'Andy what do you want?' Andy says he wants the blue pencil so the teacher says, 'Andy wants the blue pencil, give it to **him**'. The child with the blue pencil hands it over then says, 'I've given it to **him**'.

● Have a large picture of a girl and a boy and assorted clothes etc. If you use sticky-backed Velcro it will work better. Each child in turn places an item on either the girl or the boy, you can colour code if you wish to guide the choice. The player can say, 'This is **his/hers**' or 'This belongs to **him/her**', or any sentence pattern which includes the target words.

Or use the children in the group and their features and belongings.

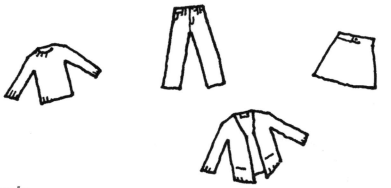

Plurals

The children may miss these out in speaking, reading and writing. These can be practised in context as above and pointed out and taught in literacy work.

● Make up a set of picture cards to illustrate different plurals: newspapers and magazines are good sources. We have a set that our younger children really like that includes one cat up one tree, two cats up one tree, two cats up two trees and one cat up two trees and other amusing combinations.

● There are plurals games produced by LDA amongst others.

● Use some of the miming games above to target plurals.

● Point out plurals in number rhymes, stories etc. Then follow up with a game of plurals. Give a word or a sentence, depending on the level at which you're working and the children have to make it a plural. As they become more confident the children can also take a turn at giving the singular starting point, or the plural could be given to be made into the singular.

Tenses

- Use pictures or the job titles of a range of occupations, such as teacher, doctor, plumber, etc. Each child in turn can mime an occupation for the others to guess. It may be helpful to practise the mimes as a group first. This can be extended to the group or individual players giving a description of a task relating to the work of an occupation using past, present and future tenses (the doctor took/is taking/will take the patient's temperature).

- Set up a daily calendar which can provide a short but regular exercise in using simple past, present and future tenses to describe personal activities. Send a simple photocopiable calendar home so parents can join in. This will also reassure and support those children who wake up not knowing what day it is nor what is likely to happen on any given day (Appendix 7).

- Use art, design, and cookery activities for memory and recall but also structure them to practise using past, present and future tenses.

- Practise tenses in prediction and retelling work during reading activities.

- Use picture sequences for story telling of what has happened, is happening and will happen next. This can be extended into story writing and, as pupils become more confident, only give the past and present, asking the pupils to put in their own ideas for the future/what will happen next.

- Passive structures need particular attention: 'The cat was chased by the mouse', is the type of sentence that trips up some pupils. It may be helpful to give or get the pupils to draw a pictorial representation; these could be literal, taken from current class work texts or fantasy (which are great fun). A set of such pictures could then be used as a 'guess the sentence' game or a game where the pupils have to ask the group questions about the drawing. Later the written sentences can be used on their own.

  Amy was following Ben.

  Jack was chased by the giant.

  The princess was caught by the dragon.

Omissions

Some children miss out words and word parts which have less stress within a phrase or sentence, such as: **a, and, the, ing, ed,** plural **s.** They may do this when speaking, reading and writing.

- If a child is persistently missing them out in his own writing *Breakthrough to Literacy* type folders can be useful. Older children can be taught to look through personal writing to check if all the appropriate words and word parts on a reference chart have been included.

- Children can use a highlighter pen and look for them in given passages. Newspaper articles are useful for this.

- They can be built into or pointed out in reading and writing tasks.

- It can also be helpful to practise tapping out the number of words in given sentences or those taken from the child's writing.

*'Him not know him not.'
(Said in disgust about his female teacher.)*

Sentences & Non-sentences

● Give and identify sentences and non-sentences about the children in the group.

Jane has brown hair – sentence

Jane brown hair – non-sentence

Then give some more, one at a time and ask children to call out sentence or non-sentence.

● As they become familiar with this use objects and/or pictures to give sentences & non-sentences about.

● **Words in a sentence.** Write down simple, monosyllabic word sentences about the children (if a child has a multi-syllabic name at first use he/she) and show them how many words are in each sentence. Show them how to put out one counter for each word, then clap the words while saying the sentence (He has brown hair – four counters). As they become familiar with this, go on to include multi-syllabic words (Amanda has long eyelashes – eight counters). Progress to saying a sentence for them to put out counters for each word, rather than show it and say it.

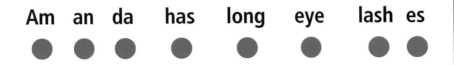

Then you can add an agreed sign/symbol for a full stop to be put at the end of each sentence and some way of indicating the capital letter – try raising hands high and saying capital and knocking on the floor whilst saying full stop.

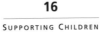

Receptive Language

Children with receptive difficulties have problems understanding even common language and may have difficulty knowing when language is directed at, or pertinent to them. They may avoid eye contact, avoid situations that they find difficult, or avoid speech – this may give the appearance of a hearing loss, so deep is the level of 'shutting off' in some children.

Avoidance, when you think about it, is a logical step to take. Since they cannot make sense of the language around them and easily become 'overloaded' with language, they shut it all out. Alternatively, they may be concentrating too hard on one word or phrase and trying to make sense of it – so that they shut out the rest.

'How are you?'
'I'm seven.'

They may look blank, pull faces, smile or giggle, cry or sulk, hide or hit out. They may carry on doing the same thing although you think you've clearly told them to stop, or do the opposite of what you say, or smile and nod – then do nothing. They may respond inappropriately because they misunderstand. They may echo or endlessly repeat what you have said, in their search for meaning.

Older children will be expected to deal successfully with more and more complex language; it may not always be apparent that they are having difficulty, or which particular structure or item of vocabulary they don't understand. As they get older, they are less willing to ask for help and learn to disguise their difficulties.

'How are you?'
'I'm Nick.'

In a busy classroom, children with receptive difficulties can easily be overlooked. They may quickly acquire a range of strategies to compensate for their lack of understanding. They may shadow another child who is in the same group and copy what she/he does. They may frequently visit the toilet, lose their books or equipment. They may have a lot of headaches or stomach-aches. They may change the subject and talk excessively about something that they are sure of. Children can become so expert at these tactics that teachers and parents are unaware of what is going on.

Whether experiencing minor or severe difficulties, such children will need direct support to listen with understanding and to follow instructions.

3

Listening and Understanding

Children with receptive difficulties have major problems with understanding and these can affect reading and writing, as well as spoken language. In all of these areas, the language used needs to be simplified. Continually check for understanding and if you suspect a difficulty:

- Repeat, 'chunking' the language with pauses to allow time for each 'chunk' to be processed.
- Simplify and re-phrase, taking out unnecessary words and explaining vocabulary.
- Ask the pupil to repeat back, in their own words, what has been said or what they are to do. In this way, understanding can be checked.
- Be ready to give more time for a child to process what has been said.

Teachers should carefully consider the language of instruction they use in lessons, giving clear explanations and being ready to repeat and/or simplify as necessary. Use visual clues to support the oral input. Build this into overall planning and practise and extend key vocabulary as part of everyday lessons.

In addition:

- Consider the position of the children concerned. Seat them where your eye falls; this is not necessarily right by you. Make sure there is enough room during carpet time. Put them where there is the least distraction.
- Verbal messages are problematical so consider putting the main message last. Messages to go home should be given last thing in the day; get the child to repeat back and always give a written note when possible. (For older children messages can be put on the board for pupils to copy.)
- Older pupils need to learn and practise self -help strategies, like acceptable ways of asking for an instruction to be repeated or to say that they have not understood. This may seem obvious but many pupils with SLI have particular difficulties with such pragmatic language skills.

Listening

Many children in mainstream and specialist settings need to develop good listening skills. There are a number of reasons why children do not seem to be good listeners.

Some children may have immature attention control and may be poor at switching from monitoring sounds to focused listening, when they need to listen for a purpose.

If we think of Reynell's stages of attention control some children of school age may still be at stage two. (See opposite.)

Child hits her own head and says, 'I can't get it, nothing is sense today.'

Teacher to child standing rigidly rooted to the spot, holding his breath. 'Are you all right?' 'I'm pulling myself together.'

'Dad was cutting the grass with a... grass scraper.'

Developmental Language Scales

Reynell, J. (1976) Developmental Language Scales NFER/Nelson

Stage 1: 0-1 year	Can pay fleeting attention but any new event will distract. Language interferes with attention.
Stage 2: 1-2 years	Will attend to own choice of activity, but will not tolerate intervention, particularly verbal. Attention is single channelled. Language interferes with attention. Must ignore other stimuli in order to concentrate on chosen activity.
Stage 3: 2-3 years	Still single channelled. Will attend to adults' choice of activity, but still difficult control. Child must stop play to attend to adults. Must listen and then shift attention back to activity with adult help.
Stage 4: 3-4 years	Single channelled, but more easily controlled. Adult verbalisation of tasks helps. Can shift attention between task and adult.
Stage 5: 4-5 years	Normal school entrant. Integrated attention for short spell. Attention span is still short. Child listens to instructions without interrupting activity to look at speaker. Child externalises language.
Stage 6: 5-6 years	Mature school entrant. Integrated attention is well controlled and sustained. Child internalises language.

Also consider that previous experiences of listening may not match school expectations.

Language at home	Language at school
Mainly conversation about the 'here and now' or about shared experiences, events and people. Not as much inferential thinking required.	Not so often about the 'here and now', more often about the past or the future and may be about new events and people. These are more likely not to be experienced at first hand. Inferential thinking required.
Tends to be more casual, with each person contributing when they have something to share or to ask.	More formalised: discussion, question and answer, following instructions.
Talking takes place in a smaller group, children getting more individual and more immediate feedback.	Takes place in a larger group, children have to take and wait their turn, less immediate feedback.
Talking takes place in a smaller group, children getting more individual and more immediate feedback.	Group identity may be poor. More likely to be group directions or questions, some children may not realise this is directed at them as part of the group.
Homes are busy and noisy places and some children may not have developed focussed listening.	Schools are busy and noisy often this is connected to activity, children are expected to listen through the noise.
Quiet may alarm them or may be linked directly with bed and sleep time i.e. time for not listening.	Children are expected to be quiet at times so that they can listen. Conversely, some children may think that being quiet is enough and may not be engaging in active listening.
May be supported by visual clues such as television, enabling the listener to pick up on information that he/she has not necessarily heard or understood. Some children may have become over reliant on visual clues.	Not always supported visually.
At home 'Listen' does not always mean that you have to listen first time, as instructions may be repeated or allowances made.	Time is precious and there's lots to do so in school pupils are expected to listen well the first time.
Comparatively short listening sessions many of which do not require a response – TV, parents' commentary.	Extended listening that usually requires a response.
May not understand what 'Listen' means but within the family allowances can be made.	In school we expect children to know what 'Listen' means. Some children need to be directly taught the sub-skills of good listening and need time and support to practise and develop these.

'No more – my brain's full.'

3

There may also be other physical, emotional or neurological difficulties.

- Hearing problems including 'Glue ear' and fluctuating hearing loss caused by hay fever, colds, etc.
- Auditory processing difficulties – difficulty perceiving and processing language. Children may have difficulty picking out from background noise or a lot of information what is relevant or pertinent to them.
- Memory difficulties.
- SLI mild or moderate.
- Have seen, seeing, waiting to see speech therapist.
- Anxiety or stress.
- ADHD.

Time spent on establishing the methods and rules for good listening within class will benefit the whole class and if a whole-school approach is taken it will benefit everyone. Such activities can be included directly as part of National Curriculum work in English (Speaking and Listening), Music and RE or PSHE and in all subject areas as part of effective class management.

First talk about what constitutes good listening, why it is necessary and how practice can improve memory and recall. Good listening helps us to:

- Learn well.
- Make friends and be a good friend.

Teacher putting papers on one side, 'I don't think I'll need these yet.' Later, she finds that Child A has put them in the bin, thinking that the teacher didn't need them at all.

Good listening can be broken down into several sub-skills:

- Good sitting – still, quiet, not fidgeting, where you can see the person who is talking.
- Good looking – at the person who is talking.
- Good thinking – listening to what is said, thinking about what is said, perhaps making a picture in your head. If it is an instruction then maybe the child needs to whisper the key words to himself until he can visualise them or think them inside his own head. (It may be necessary to describe this process to the child.)
- Taking turns – knowing when it is your turn and waiting your turn – using conversational devices such as nodding, saying 'mmmm' or 'OK'.

It is useful to include these in a whole-school policy and have picture references on view in each class (Appendix 5). These rules can be established as part of the code of conduct, and referred to and practised when necessary. It is helpful to some children (and good fun) to act out good sitting/bad sitting etc.

It is also helpful to flag up focused listening times so that those who have difficulty switching between monitoring and focused listening

3

are given an extra cue. They may also need to be addressed by name and to be shown a visual prompt. It may be helpful to briefly point out what they have to be listening for in the ensuing input, using a list or pictograms/pictures as a reminder.

Older children still need to be reminded of these but may handle the points better if they are written in a more age-appropriate way;

- Sit well (good posture, good position).
- Look regularly at the person who is talking.
- Be attentive, listen and indicate that you are listening by nodding or affirming (uh-huh, yes, no, mmmm). Make a mental picture of key points as someone is talking. Figure out the key points to note down. Unobtrusive note taking (Note taking is a skill that may need specific teaching and practice.)
- Maintain the flow of conversation/discussion by taking turns and if you wish to interrupt use an acceptable method ('Ah but, just let me say at this point.' 'I need to tell you this now before I forget'.)

It is helpful to discuss good listening in different contexts like church, canteen, yard etc. and useful to involve parents of children with speech and language difficulties since they will be able to establish good listening in home contexts.

Memory

There are different kinds of memory problems but, whatever kind of problem is involved, it is important that the child concerned is given **time** in a supportive and calm atmosphere. Acknowledge the situation and explain that many grown-ups have this problem too. Discuss the strategies below and select one to try. If it's not helping try another. This kind of approach is less likely to cause panic, or a feeling of defeat or failure and may just trigger the memory and allow the child to contribute.

Word finding

Some children have particular difficulty recalling words and need help to develop strategies to overcome this problem. We have probably all experienced this at some time, when a word is 'on the tip of our tongue' but we just can't recall it and the harder we try, the less likely it is that we will. Children with wordfinding difficulties experience this frequently. The aim is for each child to find a strategy that works and to become adept at using it independently. Try:

- Prompting with the first sound.
- Prompting with a description of the object's size, shape, colour.
- Giving the opposite: it's not black it's **** (white).
- Giving something similar: it's like a mouse it's a g**** (gerbil).

Sometimes it is difficult to use any of these if you have little idea of the word the child is trying to recall.

After intensive work on 'rough/smooth' – 'Remember we're thinking about rough and smooth'. R, picking up cheese grater and feeling it carefully, 'Yes, it's hard.'

Generally, much vocabulary work is needed. The children need to increase their vocabulary and descriptive abilities through direct labelling of objects, pictures and characters.

They need to practise various ways of defining words:

- **Category**: orange – fruit
  bus – vehicle
  pen – tool
- **Function**: orange – to be eaten
  bus – to ride on, to go on a journey on.
  pen – to write with
- **Characteristics**: orange – orange, spherical or round
  bus – lots of wheels, lots of windows, lots of seats, upstairs & downstairs, tickets
  pen – ink, nib
- **Location**: orange – fruit bowl, fruit shop, supermarket, sandwich box, tree in hot country.
  bus – road, school, bus station.
  pen – school, pencil case, shop.
- **Synonym**: orange – tangerine
  bus – coach
  pen – biro

Encourage and praise any attempt made to get meaning across. It doesn't matter what words are used e.g. 'You know, the place where we eat dinner.' 'Oh yes you mean the **hall**.' Then play some word games with school vocabulary including the word 'hall'. Later check if this word has been remembered.

- Play a game using some of the ideas given above. Start with objects in sight. 'I'm thinking of something in the classroom. It's brown, plastic and has four legs – you sit on a …' Then let the child have a turn at describing for others to guess.
- Use incomplete sentences – we cut with…., we write with…
- Use pairs – cup and …, paper and …
- Use word association. Collect as many words as possible for one given word or category – **family** – mum, dad, gran, brother, sister etc. This is a useful strategy to use at the start of a new topic in any curriculum subject to gauge what vocabulary is known. It can then be used at the end of this topic to see what vocabulary has been learned and remembered.

Short-term auditory memory

- First practise instant recall so that what is said by the leader is instantly repeated back. This can be done with instructions in class, which will have been 'chunked' for ease of understanding. It can be done for a very short time each day as an individual, paired or class activity. It can be done in the way you dismiss a class or get a class to line up. It can be done at home, or in the car if parents are involved.

- Use a child's strengths, so, if a child is musical, sing a list or if a child has good visual skills let him read the list, in words or pictures, first.
- Many children with speech and language difficulties find delivering messages problematical. This can first be practised as an instant activity within class as a sort of 'Chinese whispers' game. It can then be structured so that a child practises the message but has a written back up with him. In this way, useful techniques like mnemonics and visual imagery can be developed.
- Use some of the games below as a warm up in PE, in music sessions, in circle time, in PSHE, in literacy or in any curriculum subject wherever appropriate.

Short Term Visual Memory

Use the same principles of little and often at first. If trying to establish a sight vocabulary, for instance, have the child look at the target words for a short time every day. It is often most productive to use a multi-sensory approach and look whilst finger tracing a few times, then with eyes closed write/draw in the air or on a rough, carpeted surface. This can be a pre-cursor to a look, say, cover, write/draw technique. Some games/activities below are specifically to develop visual memory.

Long Term Auditory and Visual Memory

In many of the games below it is possible to introduce a time delay by counting to 5 or 10 before the child can carry out the activity. This is one way of making the task harder and lengthening the recall time. This should be done gradually and written or pictorial back-ups provided as prompts at first to boost confidence. Other ways to make the games more challenging include increasing the number of items used, stipulating a certain order of recall and introducing a distraction.

- It is a useful exercise to learn rhymes and poems (Appendix 3).
- Give a word at register time to be remembered, at first until break, or dinner, then all day.

The child should have regular turns at giving instructions to the others, including the adult.

- Try mnemonics with older children. If shopping for cake, apples and toothpaste the initials of the three items can be put into a word CAT (I do this all the time to remember things!). Try visual imagery – picture yourself eating a cake and an apple, then brushing your teeth! Offer different strategies to a child but help him find the one that works for him, that he can use independently. Mnemonics will not work for some children with severe and persistent memory difficulties.

Accept that there will be some children who will need to carry prompts, filofaxes or use charts and lists of key facts and vocabulary for a considerable time. Teach the use of these aids as early as possible so that they become normal practice. Jotting down things that the teacher

G. had lost his favourite scarf 'Mrs M. I can't find my neck wrapper.'

needs to remember, demonstrates and encourages the use of a small notepad as a helpful life skill that many people use.

Listening and Memory games and activities

All the vocabulary and grammar games and activities given earlier can also be used to check understanding and to develop listening skills.

- Giving instructions and following instructions can be built into lessons as an introduction or a short activity, like Music (how to play), Geography (directions), PE (directions for warm up) English (Speaking and Listening) or IT (Roamer activities).
- Allocate five or ten minutes regularly to giving instructions in class. This can be done each time children line up to leave the class e.g. 'Children with long hair line up', 'children with laces go and wash hands', 'children with short hair stand on one leg'.
- Giving Instructions. Have a leader give several instructions. The players have to listen and carry them out in order when the leader has finished speaking. Encourage the children to say the key points out loud at first, then to whisper them, then to say them silently inside their head. Start with easy ones (hop to the door) and gradually increase the length. Give simple instructions. These will have to be tailored to the level of the group but can include colours/ numbers of things or times to do an action/position/curriculum vocabulary/class equipment/clothes/people.

  For example:

- Touch something red then stand behind your chair.
- Clap two times then stand near a door.
- Point to something made of metal then stand in front of your chair.
- Hold up a ruler then put it under the table.
- If you are wearing white socks jump three times.
- Touch something made of wood then stand by a grown-up.
- Hop to the window and crawl back to your chair.
- Before you sit down clap two times.
  (NB there is a progression with before/after instructions:
  Clap your hands before you sit down (order of presentation).
  After you sit down clap your hands (order of presentation).
  Before you sit down clap your hands (Not order of presentation).
  Clap your hands after you sit down (Not order of presentation).
- Don't touch red, touch blue.
- Everyone except the children with laces stand up.
- In pairs or groups children take it in turns to give instructions for building with Lego, using multi-link, using calculators etc.
- Listen to the percussion instruments. Have two sets of percussion instruments, one set in sight and one set hidden. Children close eyes while you play one, then open their eyes and put a hand up if they can identify and play the instrument. Now send one child to the hidden set to play an instrument while the others listen and then identify and play the target instrument. The difficulty can be increased by playing two instruments and then three,

and by the children having to play the instruments in the right order.

- **Sabotage.** Set up obstacles to understanding to teach pupils that there will be times when they have to ask for clarification. Hide coats or pencils so that the children have to seek help. Have a colleague or another pupil make a noise/distraction whilst you are talking. Deliberately use words beyond that pupil's understanding. Cough or mumble part way through talking. Of course it goes without saying that it should be explained to pupils before starting, treated as a game and appropriate encouragement and rewards given. Maggie Johnson gives more ideas on this in her booklet *Active Listening*.

- **Give simple instructions**. **(Simon Says)** Let the children have three lives, then play as 'ghosts' if they lose all of them. Start by giving the Simon Says actions in a level tone and demonstrating them, giving the other – non Simon says instructions – in a different, higher tone and not doing them. As the children improve, don't demonstrate the actions.Then as they improve further, use a level tone throughout.

- **Odd One Out. Minimal Pairs.** Listen and tell the difference between minimal pair words, e.g. Man/Can Man/Map Man/Men. Initially it is probably best to use a selection that differ by first letter, then some that differ by the last letter, then by the middle letter, then a random set.

- **What's Missing?** Read a list with one thing missing – days of the week, numbers, well-known rhyme etc.

- **Listen for the word that starts with a different sound:**

apple	ant	egg	animal
boat	bat	ball	skates
car	my	coat	cow
dog	five	ditch	dad
egg	envelope	elephant	ink
fire	far	candy	feather

And so on. Later lists with one different final sound or vowel sound can be used.

- **Word/Digit repeat.** Listen and repeat back words, sentences or numbers. Start with two and when pupils are generally good at remembering those move on:

apple, orange, red, yellow, blue
dog, cat, mouse, gerbil.

(4,6)   (1,3,5)   (2,6,10,4)

I climbed.
He is tired.
She went to school.
He climbed up to the top.

Fruit Salad. Give each child round the circle the name of a fruit (colour or vehicle or animal) in sets of three – apple, banana, orange, apple, banana, orange (If you have a larger group adjust the number of names accordingly – have 5 or 6 – apple, orange, banana, lemon, pear, grape.)

Establish rules – walking carefully, no bumping, into middle and out to a different place. Then play the game where the ones you call swap places, so if you call 'apples, oranges' they swap and if you call 'bananas, oranges' they swap and if you call 'fruit salad' everybody swaps.

- **Using a calculator.** Ask the children to key in numbers; start with 2 and work up to 5 or 6. Say the numbers for the children to remember. They enter them in, then show you the numbers.
- **Multi-link.** The children have their hands in their laps while you say two colours (start with two and work up to five or six). The children remember and pick up the colours and hide them in their hands until everyone's done, then you check. When they've got used to the routine they can take turns choosing/giving colours.
- Each child has 10 multilink, one of each colour.
  Join a red one and a blue one.
  Join red, blue, green.
  Join all except the blue and green…
- Give each child a multilink cube, some can have the same colours.
  Reds stand.
  Reds and greens change places
  Reds and blues stand; greens and yellows lie down.
  If you have red clap 2 times…
- **Giving Clues.** The children take it in turns to give three clues about a picture while the others listen and decide what it is. To check for good listening ask children at the end what clues have been given. The use of pictures keeps children on track and ensures that they don't change their minds halfway through.
- **Pairs.** Working in pairs, the children ask each other about a given subject and then report back to the group (their partner's favourite food, drink, colour, number, game, TV programme, pets, brother's and sister's names…).
- **Listen for a category.** The children have to repeatedly stand up or sit down as they hear a word from a given category. Name the category then read in a level voice, or tape record and play back while joining in or observing. It is easier with two adults, one to read in a level tone and the other to monitor what the children do. So if the named category is 'food', the children stand, sit, stand, and sit as they hear each food word. (If preferred the children can raise and lower their arms instead.) For example, red, **apple**, skirt, one, cat, knife, green, **toast**, horse, mum, nine, **baked beans** etc.

● **Say and ask.** Tell the children what category they are listening for – vehicles, for example. Read each group of four then ask, 'What vehicles did I say?'

NB Use the list this way first so the target words are the last ones. Then try reversing the list so the target words are said first and have to be remembered longer.

apple	banana	car	bus
orange	yellow	lorry	train
elephant	giraffe	boat	hovercraft
four	five	bike	plane

Use lists of words that begin with the same sound, category lists, vocabulary lists, linked to particular subject areas, random numbers.

Tell a simple one or two sentence 'story' and ask a question about it. As children become familiar with this, lengthen the sentences and/or ask more questions or make them inferential.
A boy called Tom went to the park and played on the swing.
Who went to the park? What did he play on?
I went to Chester on the bus.
Where did I go? How did I get there?
I had my tea at Carol's house.
Where did I eat? What meal did I have?
The next day my sister and I went to town.
When did they go? Where did they go? Who went to town?
My sister said, 'I'm helping Mum to clear up'.
Who is helping Mum? What are they doing? Who is speaking?

● **Describe one child in minute detail.** Child concerned stands up if they think it's them; others put their hands up if they know who it is. (NB Children need to become aware when they have been given enough information to make a good guess.)
I'm thinking of someone who has white socks.
I'm thinking of someone who has white socks and blue eyes.
I'm thinking of someone who has white socks, blue eyes and brown hair.
I'm thinking of someone who has white socks, blue eyes and long, brown hair.

● **Listening and drawing, circling, colouring**… Photocopiable sheets and on cassette (see resources list).

● **Whisper game.** Have children close their eyes or sit round with you in the middle. Whisper their names for them to line up at the door ready to move on. If they get good at this make it harder – whisper initials or descriptions or simply look directly at each child in turn to signal that they are to line up.

● **Kim's Game.** A number of items are placed on a tray or table. Choose a set pertinent to current work e.g. fabric, glass, wood, metal, plastic items when covering 'materials'. The child or children are given a chance to look at them, then they turn away and close their eyes.

One item is removed and this has to be named after a second look at the tray. The number of items removed can gradually be increased. Or use a magazine picture which has lots of detail, look at it then cover it and try to remember as many items as you can.

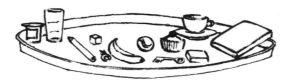

- **Traffic Police.** Make up some car number plates on paper or card. One player is the robber who moves a number across the table; the policeman has to look carefully at it. The robber hides the number and the policeman has to write it down or radio it to headquarters.

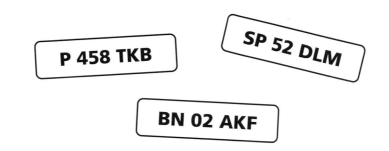

- **Jigsaws.** Teach the child a system, so he is looking for pieces that fit together by colour, shape, parts of objects and edge and middle pieces. Then try to complete it using shape alone, by turning the jigsaw over onto its plain, reverse side.

Supportive signing

It may be helpful to consider using a supportive signing system that runs alongside spoken language. Communication is obviously difficult for our children whether they have a severe speech production difficulty, a receptive difficulty or an expressive difficulty. But many children have well-developed visual skills and respond well to staff using mime and gesture.

Paget Gorman Signed Speech (PGSS) has been specifically designed for use with children with speech and language impairment. It is not a language in its own right but accompanies talk. Paget is a very logical system based on a number of hand shapes and basic signs that are linked to class groups like, animals, vehicles, food, etc. It is also possible to sign all grammatical markers such as plurals, tense endings, possessives, etc. It can be used to:

- introduce and support the acquisition of specific vocabulary and language concepts
- introduce and support the acquisition of specific grammatical terms
- encourage children to include all necessary words in an utterance
- slow down speech in children who rush their talk and push all

their words together
- assist decoding during reading without verbally interrupting the reader

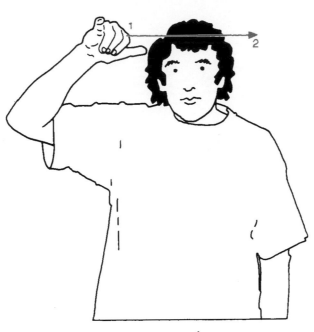

aeroplane

In addition, Cued Articulation, a signing system designed particularly to assist children with speech production, has proved extremely useful when working with children with speech production difficulties. It enables us to cue them in to a particular sound in a way that is low key and yet reminds them how to shape their tongue and lips and how to form the sound. Paget and Cued Articulation may not be suitable for all educational settings but it may be worthwhile to explore available systems and ways of visually cueing and supporting children with speech and language difficulties.

Social Use of Language Skills and Behaviour

The playground can be a frightening, lonely place.

Many children with speech and language impairment are unable to interpret their peers' colloquial language, jokes, nuances and implied meanings and this impedes the development of social relationships and making friends. They can be really lonely and ready targets for bullying, yet unable to use language to explain their predicament accurately or to resolve the conflict. They may use inappropriate behaviour if they have poor understanding of body language, gesture, greetings and acceptable forms of address.

Some of these difficulties are to do with what are termed 'pragmatic language skills'; these are bound up in the culture and customs of society, family and friends. They are the sorts of skills that are very hard to teach, and most of us learn them as we go along. For example, knowing that it is more acceptable to say 'Good morning', to a teacher rather than 'Hiya, how ya doin?' Or that whilst it is acceptable to say 'Good night' several times to the same people, initially when you go to bed, later when you come back down for the book you've forgotten and later still to get a drink…that in the morning you only say 'Good morning' once to each person.

Pupils with poor social language skills may be the pupils whose names are mentioned frequently in staffrooms, as teachers, other adults and peers may interpret their responses in a range of negative ways. Such pupils may:

- 'switch off' during lessons because they have very poor listening and understanding skills
- be restless, fidgety and may shout out
- have difficulty following instructions
- appear unconcerned if they forget to bring things from home
- answer rather strangely using the wrong words or a literal interpretation
- be noticed a lot at play times because they are more 'physical' than other children, in because of their inability to communicate in the normal way
- be socially immature and have co-ordination problems
- have difficulties remembering names, following games, joining in with chatter
- often be on their own or complaining that no-one will play with them
- seem to be 'saying and doing it on purpose'.

Younger children will need help to develop play skills; ring games have proved most useful and can be readily adapted. (There are a number of books which have a selection of playground games, listed in the Books and Resources section.) In Acton Park Infants School we have a whole school system that supports all children. We actively teach ring games and then reward children for playing these. Each child has a 100 square playground chart and at breaktimes duty staff give out stickers to be stuck on these charts. The children are rewarded in a weekly service for each set of ten stickers earned. This has worked well as all the children have knowledge of the same games and it is both easier for them to join and follow games and for staff to prompt and encourage good play. Incidentally, this system has also developed maths skills: all the children know how many stickers they have and their ability to count in tens quickly improves! In the summer, we use a range of equipment designed to be fun but also effective in developing motor skills as well as social skills (French skipping, large noughts and crosses, skipping ropes, target hoopla games). I have found it helpful to spend some additional time teaching my pupils the ring games and use of the playtime equipment so they are more confident at playtimes.

Some children find peer group jargon and social situations especially difficult because they interpret language absolutely literally. This can be addressed directly by collecting, explaining and using common colloquial expressions and sayings; for example phrases used by adults like 'Pull your socks up', and 'Jump to it'. These can be found in written materials and they can be directly linked to topic work. In addition, take note of those expressions in current vogue such as 'Wicked', 'Monstrous' or 'Cool'. Similarly, slightly older children can explore and collect different kinds of jokes and puns. It has proved useful for older children to learn to recognise such language for themselves. They can report statements that sound odd or nonsensical, discuss and possibly collect them for reference. A few years ago 'well bad' was much in use in the playground – a trial for those children who literally interpret and for whom it didn't make sense.

Flat speech, with no intonation and little or no expression, can also be a characteristic linked to difficulties with understanding and with being understood. Speaking with expression can be demonstrated in the activities above and can also be demonstrated and practised whilst reading and through role-play and drama. It has proved helpful to discuss and explore body language, ways of speaking with different expression, greetings and partings as discrete skills and then to practise these.

- **How are you feeling?** In my class we have a feelings board and each morning the children consider how they are feeling and put their name by the appropriate label – happy/sad/worried/full of beans/excited/tired. This provides a short opportunity to discuss why we have put our names by a particular label. We have now developed this to discussing some ways we can 'wake up' children

Mr M used to tap his watch and say 'What time do you call this?' when a pupil was late. When Mr M himself was late G leapt to his feet, tapped his watch and said very loudly, 'What time do you call this?'

who are feeling tired or 'out of sorts'. Our list includes a snack, a drink, short period of exercise in the fresh air, washing face or brain gym. Of course at first the children invariably chose the first two. Sometimes these worked but often did not, that is they were still not settling and tackling work well, so I was able to comment on this and steer them towards trying the other strategies.

This activity enables us to teach the vocabulary and concepts of emotions and also to raise the children's level of awareness in line with Sensory Integration ideas. We use some brain gym ideas coupled with short energising techniques and relaxation techniques first thing in the morning after looking at our feelings board but also throughout the day. These are also especially useful after play and dinner breaks.

I have one or two children who find it very difficult to sit still for any length of time so I try to stretch and move the whole group every now and then but also have some other agreed procedures.

- **Moving breaks**. A child is allowed to have a quiet walk round, look out of the window for a few moments, walk to toilets and wash hands and come back; that is stretch their legs for a short time. We practised this and talked about it a lot before it became an established and non-disruptive routine and it certainly seems to help.
- **'Brain gym'**. This is intended wake up the brain, and my children like this. There are various exercises that are supposed to stimulate thinking. Here are three:
  Rub ear lobes then roll them up and down.
  Draw large sideways figure eights in the air, right hand, then left hand then both hands together. (If you teach the children to keep their heads still but track their thumb nail with their eyes only, this doubles as a visual tracking exercise.)
  Energy yawn – massage muscles where lower jaw meets upper jaw in front of ear. This invariably makes you yawn which you enjoy. Then take an energising breath – place hands on table, or if standing, loosely by sides. Lower chin to chest, relax/make shoulders floppy, feel the gentle stretch in the back of the neck. Take a deep slow breath in through nose whilst gently lifting chin up and then putting head back, allowing back to arch slightly and so opening rib cage. Then exhale through mouth whilst curving the back and bringing chin back to rest on chest. A couple of these are a real wake up.
- **Mini relaxation**. Standing or sitting straight and tall but relaxed/ floppy shoulders, arms, hands. (It can help to teach the children to put their hands loosely together or to put finger and thumb loosely together with other fingers curled.) Close eyes and take three slow, but very quiet breaths in through nose and out through mouth with a quiet sigh.

4

Behaviour

Every school needs to have a well-established and clearly understood discipline and bullying policy in place. This should include:

- Clear rules and routines within a climate of mutual respect and clear expectations.
- Clear system of rewards and sanctions, including a time-out 'thinking' area in class and a time-out system for beyond the classroom.
- Attractive and well-organised environment with adequate resources for differentiated curriculum.
- A set of procedures including tactical ignoring, reminders of rules, questioning, giving choices, direction, warnings, redirecting to defuse a situation, using time out, setting up personal behaviour agreements if necessary and using a team approach to solving persistent behaviour problems.

However, some children with SLI and with other impairments will need more than this. They may need to understand what is **not** acceptable alongside what **is** acceptable. They may need to practise acceptable behaviours. With unacceptable behaviours we have found it necessary to state their unacceptability, firmly but calmly, then to demonstrate what would be acceptable in that situation. This usually needs thinking through carefully, as most children will follow the examples given literally.

Different situations require different behaviours and some children will need re-teaching for each new location or each new set of circumstances. Using the principles of Carol Gray's *Social Stories*, we also write personal books for some children, addressing particular behaviour and use them to teach and then to be read to, and by the children.

It has proved helpful with older children to further explore a range of strategies for breaks and lunchtimes. Discuss the rules and procedures for these times. Discuss strategies for joining a group, leaving a group and possible responses to peer group language. Discuss possible strategies for dealing with teasing and bullying: it will help if each child has a plan ready to use. Again it is most helpful if this is approached as a whole-school issue, with procedures in place for all. However, pupils with social language difficulties will need additional, direct teaching on how to respond, behave appropriately and keep safe in a range of situations. At school much of this work can be carried out with peers through circle time activities, drama and role-play.

Discuss with the pupil(s) how in some situations they will not understand what is meant and will not be able to make themselves understood. Discuss possible strategies:

- 'I'm not very good with words'/'I don't understand'/'Could you write it down please?'
- 'Can you tell me another way please?'

- 'I'll just leave it for now thank you.'
- Phone home for help. Teach them to always check that they have money and/or a pre-paid phone card for the phone. As a back-up teach them how to make a reverse charge call.
- Sometimes in peer group situations it may be best to walk away. If appropriate, AFASIC produce a smart, unobtrusive plastic card that briefly but clearly explains the holder's difficulties with language. (There are a number of books with ideas for activities in the Books and Resources section, including Wendy Rinaldi's *Social Use of Language Programme*.) Interventions are most effective if parents are involved as well, contributing to a united approach by school and home, and it may also be useful for children to attend out-of-school clubs like Rainbows, Beavers, Gymnastics or Swimming.

Personal organisation, or lack of it, can have a significant impact on children's ability to cope in the classroom, and therefore on their resulting behaviour. It is important for teachers to 'catch them being good', to explicitly teach and reward good organisation:

- At the table, organising books, pencil, personal dictionary, ruler etc, including getting them out and putting them away.
- Taking care of own belongings – book bag, PE kit, sandwich box etc.
- Taking responsibility for specific jobs around class.
- Remembering to bring in items needed for art or other curriculum work.

There are some simple items that may make life easier for older children and points which parents can be made aware of:

- A smart notebook, a filofax, a very small cassette recorder or electronic organiser – whatever is 'in vogue' – in which to jot things that may otherwise be forgotten such as messages for parents or homework, party invitations, trips, etc. It can also contain vital information like personal addresses, phone numbers and emergency plans for who to phone and where to go when things go wrong.
- Instead of parents remembering and packing games kit, swimming kit, etc. children should learn to do so themselves. Have a weekly timetable in a conspicuous place that is checked at a regular time every day. Pack school bags the evening before after checking the timetable.
- Suggest that parents buy a talking watch for children with difficulties understanding time. These are available from The RNIB, PO Box 173, Peterborough, PE2 6WS.
- Lack of awareness of possible difficulties and dangers make road safety training an absolute priority for teachers and parents. RoSPA has some very useful resources.
- It is useful to have a basic tool kit for school. This might include pens, felts, calculator, inhaler, etc. and it should be the child's responsibility to organise replacements. Sometimes it is helpful to have two, one for home and homework and one for school.

	Sunday	Monday	Tuesday	Wednesday	Thursday	Friday	Saturday
1		1	1	1	1	1	
2		2	2	2	2	2	
3		3	3	3	3	3	
4		4	4	4	4	4	
5		5	5	5	5	5	
		At home	At home	At home	At home	At home	
		Do homework for:	Do homework for:	Do homework for:	Do homework for:	Do homework for:	
Pack swimming kit		Pack PE kit	Pack PE kit	Collect materials for D+T	Pack Karate kit	Pack PE kit	Make sure all sports kit and school uniform is washed
Check that all homework is done							
Dinner money							
Bus fare/pass							

Developmental Co-ordination Difficulties

Some children with speech and language impairment also have co-ordination difficulties, sometimes termed Dyspraxia or Developmental Co-ordination Difficulties (DCD). Like speech and language impairment, DCD encompass a range of problems:

    D irection
    E mbarrassment
    V isual perception
m **E** mory, listening
    L aterality
    O ral motor skills
    P lanning, proprioception, pain
    M ovement
    E motion (impulsive or low arousal levels)
    N ormal intelligence
    T actile system affected
    A uditory processing, attention
re **L** ationships

(With kind permission of Amanda Hopkin, Head Paediatric Occupational Therapist, Maelor Children's Centre, Wrexham)

This is a wide-ranging list that incorporates sensory integration difficulties. The overlap with SLI can clearly be seen and so some of the areas affected have already been covered. In addition, the vestibular and the proprioceptive systems may be working inefficiently. The vestibular system is the processing of information on gravity and balance through the inner ear. The proprioceptive system is the processing of information about body parts and body position through muscles, ligaments and nerves.

Some children may have an inefficient sensory intake and therefore actively seek extra sensory stimulation. Such children are moving and fidgeting all the time, they fiddle with things and may often end up breaking them. They act impulsively and tend to get messy with food or paint, and their clothes become twisted and untucked, though they will probably not notice this at all.

Conversely, some children may routinely take in too much sensory information and so avoid sensory stimuli. These children may not walk up and down stairs confidently, they dislike climbing frames and slides, are easily overwhelmed by movement and may well be travel-sick. They may avoid certain smells and tastes in foods and may be picky eaters.

5

If these difficulties are severe then advice can be sought from the Physiotherapy Service or Occupational Therapy Service. They may be able to offer some physiotherapy sessions and, if appropriate, a programme. However, many therapy services are over-stretched and less severe problems can be targeted regularly in school both in discrete sessions and as a warm up in PE. Short, regular sessions have proved successful for some children. We take a whole-school approach to this at Acton Park Infants School, and pupils from mainstream classes join in with some from the language class to follow a daily exercise programme. This programme is described on page 40-46. Parents can supervise or join in with some exercises and can encourage ball play, skipping, bike riding etc. Some children benefit greatly from attending swimming, golf, gym or dance clubs.

Fine motor

Some children also have fine motor difficulties and generally need extra practice at threading, cutting, tracing, painting etc. These can usually be fitted in to the school day at primary level; short, regular sessions have proved most successful. Activities can be practised at home too.

- Encourage short, daily finger-flexing exercises, there are a number of these in our motor programme given below. It is most useful to do some of these before a writing session.
- Offer a range of pens and pencils.
- Pencil grips and, for older children, triangular shaped pencils can help. ('Tri-go' is LDA's latest pencil grip and it is an excellent design.)
- Cardboard, finger-shaped finger spaces with a dab of blutack on the back can be used to help establish good spacing. They eventually become redundant.
- Offer a range of scissors – left and right-handed, spring-loaded and very sharp for cutting fabric.
- A sloped desktop that fits on school tables is useful. Construct one from a file or purchase one from a number of suppliers. For older children there are some that fit discreetly into an A4 folder.
- Provide active demonstration of, and then regular practice at, good sitting at a table. We have a short chant – bottom back, feet flat (and hands in your lap). Posture cushions are very helpful for some children and there is a range available. (Movin'sit from Gymnic, is triangular and fits neatly onto school chairs. It has a raised, knobbly surface which really helps those children with proprioceptive difficulties as they can move about more discreetly.) Some children will then need footrests so that their feet can be flat. These can be simply made from telephone directories or catalogues.Establish the correct positioning for right and left-handers.
- Set up and encourage or direct the use of a hand gym with things like bubble wrap to pop, pegs and bulldog clips to open and shut, multi-link and pop-it beads to fix together.
- Use a handwriting system and recognise that some children will need daily practice, then regular practice for a lot longer than other children. Older children may find paper with raised marker

38

lines helpful (available from Philip and Tacey). Some children may also respond better to cursive script and to pen, rather than pencil or to using a keyboard. Keyboards are cumbersome for note taking in class however, and it is more successful to have lesson notes provided for some children who then use the keyboard to re-draft these and make them their own.

- Teach simple folk dances which are good fun, develop listening skills, a sense of rhythm and are a way of learning and practising using right and left hands. I give our young children a ponytail band to put on their right wrist to help them remember which is their right hand. (A range of folk dance music that comes with instructions is available from Folk in Education, details in the Books and Resources section.)

Motor skills development programme

Plan to have a short session of about ten minutes each day if possible, or at least twice a week. The following sets of exercises are a guide. Obviously, staff need to assess their pupil's current performance and difficulties and then draw up an appropriate programme. This set of exercises starts at crawling and not all groups will need to start at this basic level. Be flexible and respond to the progress the children are making, particular difficulties and also to moods, (theirs and yours). I tend to use the same set of exercises for at least a week, but sometimes longer. My mainstream colleague likes to work at one or two tasks exclusively until progress is evident. There are many ways of organising the sessions. We use the school hall at changeover times for the ten minutes when it is not in use while PE or other classes are changing or getting organised, so there is no infringement of precious hall times. If the weather is good, we go outside in the fresh air and also to use the concrete steps to walk up and down.

Establish a routine for starting and finishing the session; I tend to keep the same one for several weeks. Our current beginning routine is standing relaxation. Good Standing (straight and tall, feet slightly apart, eyes open, arms loosely down by sides and feel as if there's a string tied to the top of the head gently pulling you tall and straight) with eyes closed and breathing quietly in through nose and out through mouth, three breaths. Our current ending routine is Good Standing, then walking out of the hall either on toes or on heels, children choose which way.

An alternative is: Good standing, then flop forwards from the waist like a floppy doll, dangle for a few seconds then uncurl back to upright. Good standing, shake hands vigorously. Slowly and carefully drop head to one shoulder, hold, roll head back to midpoint, hold, drop head to other shoulder, hold and back to midpoint. Gently roll head round. Good standing, hands holding sides at bottom of ribcage, breathe in through nose and out through mouth, finishing with a deep breath in and out. Good standing, shake hands vigorously.

5

Relaxation techniques both sitting and lying down, can also be used as a finishing routine. Good sitting, legs crossed, back straight but not tense, then chin tipped down to throat, eyes closed and back of wrists on knees, fingers loosely curled, quiet breathing. Lying on back, legs slightly apart, hands down by sides, palms up, fingers loosely curled, eyes closed.

It is important when finishing with relaxation to 'wake the body up' before moving back to class: shake arms, legs one at a time, then whole body, then stretch up.

We assess in an ongoing manner by observing children each day in the sessions and in and around school. We update the record sheets more precisely about once a term by going through the activities and noting down how each child is doing. A sample record sheet is given in this pack.

In our specialist language class we also use PE warm-up times to practise the above skills. We carry out the hand and finger exercises regularly in class before writing and have a shoe box 'hand gym' that the children use in class. We also incorporate rhythm, clapping and tapping exercises in our music and listening activities and a range of manipulative skills within class work. All of these complement the work carried out in the daily exercise sessions.

Daily tasks

Repeat each exercise 3, 5, or 10 times as appropriate and as time allows.

A
1. Starting routine.
2. In prone position, lying flat on stomach, arms bent with elbow to palm flat on floor, hands level with shoulders. Lie straight. Lift head slowly, hold, then slowly lower.
3. As 2. Lift head and top of trunk.
4. On hands and knees hold balance then rock back onto heels and forward again.
5. Good crawling.
6. Creeping on hands and feet.
7. Stand straight and tall, put arms out sideways at shoulder level, spin round then stand and gain balance. If steady, can try with eyes closed.
8. Stand straight and tall, with (L) hand touch (R) shoulder, elbow, knee, foot and then with (R) hand touch (L) shoulder, elbow, knee, foot.
9. Finishing routine.

B
1. Starting routine.
2. As 2. above but lift head and top of trunk but this time fully extend arms and hold gaze straight ahead for count of 3, then 5.
3. Lie straight in prone position then roll onto back and hold, roll onto stomach and hold.
4. As 4. above but then roll over and over.
5. In prone position pull forward, stretching one arm to reach forward then the other.
6. On hands and knees hold balance then rock back onto heels and forward again, then good crawling.
7. Stand straight and tall, put arms out sideways at shoulder level, spin round, then stand and gain balance. If steady, can try with eyes closed.
8. Stand straight and tall, with (L) hand touch (R) shoulder, elbow, knee, foot and then with (R) hand touch (L) shoulder, elbow, knee, foot.
9. Finishing routine.

C

1. Starting routine.
2. As 2. above. Lift head and top of trunk but this time fully extend arms and hold gaze straight ahead for count of 5.
3. Lie straight in prone position, then roll onto back and hold, roll onto stomach and hold.
4. As 4. above.
5. In prone position pull forward, stretching one arm to reach forward, then the other, then good crawling.
6. On hands and knees hold balance, then rock back onto heels and forward again.
7. Stand straight and tall, put arms out sideways at shoulder level, spin round then stand and gain balance. If steady, can try with eyes closed.
8. Stand straight and tall, with (L) hand touch (R) shoulder, elbow, knee, foot and then with (R) hand touch (L) shoulder, elbow, knee, foot.
9. Finishing routine.

D

1. Starting routine.
2. Lie on back, straight and flat with head in midline position. Slowly and carefully roll head from side to middle to other side, holding in each position.
3. Lie on back, straight and flat with head in midline position. Bend (R) knee to chest, holding knee to chest. Then (L) knee.
4. Straighten (R), then (L), and then both legs vertically, hold, then slowly lower.
5. Roll over and over, then balance on hands and knees before good crawling.
6. Stand straight and tall, with (L) elbow touch (R) knee and then with (R) elbow touch (L) knee.
7. Eyes closed touch body parts as Teacher calls them out.
8. Eyes closed lift/raise body parts as Teacher calls them out.
9. Finishing routine.

E

1. Starting routine.
2. Lie on back, straight and flat with head in midline position. Slowly and carefully roll head from side to middle to other side, holding in each position.
3. Lie on back, straight and flat with head in midline position. Bend (R) knee to chest, holding knee to chest. Then (L) knee.
4. Straighten (R) leg and (R) arm vertically, hold then slowly lower, then (L) and then both. Now raise both and (R) hand holding (R) foot, (L) hand holding (L) foot so hold feet, arms and legs vertical and balance.
5. Roll over and over, then good crawling.
6. Stand straight and tall, with (L) elbow touch (R) knee and then with (R) elbow touch (L) knee.
7. Eyes closed touch body parts as Teacher calls them out.
8. Eyes closed lift/raise body parts as Teacher calls them out.
9. Finishing routine.

F

1. Starting routine.
2. Good standing, then holding a good position good walking.
3. Walk on toes forwards and then backwards.
4. Walk on heels forwards then backwards.
5. Lie on back, straight and flat with head in midline position. Bend (R) knee to chest, holding knee to chest. Then (L) knee.
6. Straighten (R) leg and (R) arm vertically, hold then slowly lower, then (L) and then both. Now raise both and (R) hand holding (R) foot, (L) hand holding (L) foot so hold feet, arms and legs vertical and balance.
7. Eyes closed lift/raise body parts as Teacher calls them out.
8. Good standing touch tip of (R) index/pointing finger to tip of nose then (L) index/pointing finger to tip of nose. Repeat with eyes closed. Then touch tip of (R) index/pointing finger to (L) shoulder, elbow, knee and vice versa, eyes open then eyes closed.
9. Finishing routine.

5

G

1. Starting routine.
2. Good standing, then holding a good position good walking, stop to adult direction.
3. Walk on toes forwards and then backwards. Now good standing go into a balance on toes, bend knees and sink into a toe squat balance and gently bounce before rising to standing again. Try to have no hands touching floor. If it helps press hands to thighs,
4. Walk on heels forwards then backwards.
5. Lie on back, straight and flat with head in midline position. Bend (R) knee to chest, holding knee to chest. Then (L) knee.
6. Straighten (R) leg and (R) arm vertically, hold then slowly lower, then (L) and then both. Now raise both and (R) hand holding (R) foot, (L) hand holding (L) foot so hold feet, arms and legs vertical and balance.
7. Eyes closed lift/raise body parts as Teacher calls them out.
8. Good standing, touch tip of (R) index/pointing finger to tip of nose, then (L) index/pointing finger to tip of nose. Repeat with eyes closed. Then touch tip of (R) index/pointing finger to (L) shoulder, elbow, knee and vice versa, eyes open, then eyes closed.
9. Finishing routine.

H

1. Starting routine.
2. High balance on knees, legs stretched out behind with top of feet flat on floor, arms down by sides. Hold. Then raise arms to shoulder height and bring to front of body with palms together, hold. Then turn hands so backs of hands are together so can move arms back, trying to keep them level, then forwards again returning to front.
3. High balance on knees then sink down, then stretch arms out in front along the floor, palms flat to floor, head between arms, gaze down to floor. Hold then return to sunken position, then to high kneeling.
4. Curl up small, then roll over and over curled up.
5. Good standing, then holding a good position good walking, stop to adult direction.
6. Walk on heels forwards then backwards. Walk on insides of feet then outsides of feet. Walk on toes forwards and then backwards. Now good standing, go into a balance on toes, bend knees and sink into a toe squat balance and gently bounce before rising to standing again. Try to have no hands touching floor. If it helps press hands to thighs,
7. Good standing, (R) hand to (L) knee three times, then (L) hand to (R) knee three times.
8. Good standing, then fold arms and keep them folded so they don't touch the floor, cross legs at ankles and sink down to sitting. Hold good sitting with legs crossed, back straight, neck tall, then keeping arms folded, swing legs round to side, go to kneeling then to standing.
9. Finishing routine.

I

1. Starting routine.
2. High balance on knees, legs stretched out behind with top of feet flat on floor, arms down by sides. Hold. Then raise arms to shoulder height and bring to front of body with palms together, hold. Then turn hands so backs of hands are together so can move arms back, trying to keep them level, then forwards again returning to front.
3. High balance on knees then sink down, then stretch arms out in front along the floor, palms flat to floor, head between arms, gaze down to floor. Hold then return to sunken position, then to high kneeling.
4. Curl up small then roll over and over curled up.
5. Good standing, then holding a good position, good walking. Stop to adult direction. Try this with running/jogging.
6. Good standing, then quiet jumping, bending knees as land, good standing and two quiet breaths, then bend one leg raising knee to waist height and balance for count of 3 or 5 then lower leg. Repeat all this, then balance on other leg. (Aim for balance to a count of 10; count down for children at first i.e. 5,4,3,2,1 then let them do this themselves.)
7. Good standing, (R) hand to (L) knee three times, then (L) hand to (R) knee three times.
8. Good standing, then fold arms and keep them folded, cross legs at ankles and sink down to sitting. Hold good sitting with legs crossed, back straight, neck tall, keeping arms folded swing legs round to side, go to kneeling then to standing.
9. Finishing routine.

5

J

1. Starting routine.
2. Balance on bottom with legs held diagonally straight up in front and hands straight in front towards legs.
3. Slide across floor on back then on stomach. Walk on bottom with legs out in front, hands on thighs or hips, stretching one leg forward at a time so 'walking' not sliding.
4. Good standing, then good jumping with legs bending at knees on landing, on spot then sustained jumping round room. Repeat with hopping.
5. Walk heel to toe. At first children will probably look at feet to check that the heel touches the toes each time, aim for good standing/good walking without looking at feet.
6. Good standing then standing twist. Hands on hips keep legs still and rotate trunk right round to (R) and then (L).
7. Good standing, then keeping legs still, bend trunk forwards, backwards, to either side.
8. Cat's got measles (good standing, then jump and cross legs at ankles, then jump apart).
9. Finishing routine.

K

1. Starting routine.
2. Balance on one hand and one leg then on other hand and other leg. Balance on bottom.
3. Slide across floor on back then on stomach. Walk on bottom with legs out in front, hands on thighs or hips, stretching one leg forward at a time so 'walking' not sliding.
4. Good standing then good jumping with legs bending at knees on landing, on spot then sustained jumping round room. Repeat with hopping.
5. Walk heel to toe. At first children will probably look at feet to check that the heel touches the toes each time. Aim for good standing/good walking without looking at feet.
6. Standing twist, then keeping legs still bend trunk forwards, backwards, to either side.
7. Cat's got measles (good standing, then jump and cross legs at ankles, then jump apart).
8. Good standing, arms stretched out in front move them round until stretched out sideways at shoulder level, then up above head, then reverse until back in front stretch.
9. Finishing routine.

L

1. Starting routine.
2. Balance on different parts of body as Teacher calls them out – one leg, other leg, bottom, one leg and one arm…
3. Balance on one hand and walk round that hand, repeat with other hand.
4. Good standing, balance on one leg and swing other leg forwards and backwards, then draw circles in air with flexed foot. Do this on other side.
5. Sitting bridge. Good long sitting, legs stretched out in front and hands on thighs, then put hands flat on floor level with waist and fingers pointing forwards. Push down on hands and heels and raise bottom off floor, keeping legs diagonally straight, look at toes.
6. Cross lateral. Good standing then stretch (R) arm and (R) leg forward and hold, repeat with (L) arm & leg saying "same side". Next try (R) arm and (L) leg stretched forward and then (L) arm and (R) leg, saying "opposite sides".
7. Good standing. Shoulder stretching, keeping rest of body still raise both shoulders and lower, then one shoulder at a time. Push shoulders forwards and backwards then rotate them.
8. Good standing. Stretch arms in front then to sides and up as before, then keeping rest of body still windmill/rotate both arms, then rotate one arm at a time. Then scissor arms at sides and then in front of body, close but not touching.
9. Finishing routine.

We also have sessions using balls and beanbags for throwing, catching, rolling, spinning, dribbling etc and if appropriate, we work directly on learning our (R) and (L) hand, though this is often left to KS 2.

5

Assessment

(This will probably take more than one session.)

1. Starting routine.

2. As teacher calls them out move in various ways – good walking, walk on toes, heels, heel to toe, jump, hop etc, stopping when teacher calls stop.

3. Balancing on various body parts for count down from 10 (one leg, each leg in turn, bottom, hand and leg, knees…)

4. Rocking. Standing, sway from side to side and forwards and backwards. Lying on back rock from side to side. On knees sway from side to side and forwards and backwards.

5. Children choose to sit or lie down and with eyes closed touch body parts as teacher calls them out quite quickly.

6. With ball throw and catch, bounce and catch, dribble and stop with foot.

7. With bean bag move from hand to hand in front, over and under each leg in turn, over shoulder to other hand then up and round front back to first hand, eyes open then eyes closed.

8. Cross lateral. Crawling, creeping on hands and feet, opposite arm and leg stretched out in front, (R) hand to (L) shoulder, elbow, knee, toe and vice versa and Cat's got the measles (good standing, then jump and cross legs at ankles, then jump apart).

9. Finishing routine.

(See record sheet on page 46.)

Hand and finger exercises

If appropriate, I try to establish the habit of using dominant hand first in these exercises, so right-handers will use right hand first and left-handers use left hand first. This is difficult with young children who have no secure understanding of right and left so I use 'pencil hand and not pencil hand or 'band hand' and 'other hand' to begin with.

1. Establish good sitting, with chair close enough to table, sitting back in chair with feet flat on floor. Shrug, then rotate shoulders to relax posture. Shake arms down by sides.

2. Palms together, fingers spread, press fingers together and push elbows out with heel of hands down.

3. Fingers interlaced, stretch both arms in front and push palms forwards.

4. Monkey Grip – interlock fingers of one hand with the fingers of the other hand. Pull apart for 5 seconds then release for 5 seconds. Repeat 3–5 times.

5. Open and close fingers, stretching them on the open movement.

6. Make a fist of each hand, then vigorously flick fingers out.

7. Slowly curl fingers closed, then slowly curl them open.

8. Fingers curled point with each finger in turn, right hand then left hand.

9. Typing/Piano playing – both hands with forearms resting on table. The typewriter keys/ piano keys need to be hit quite hard with separate fingers.

10. Paper scrunch – start with tissue and then try newspaper or other paper that requires more strength. Start at one corner with the writing hand; gather all the paper into a tight ball. Throw it into the bin for target practice.

11. Move the pencil – hold pencil in the air, with the writing hand, grasping it at one end. Try to wriggle the hand up to the other end of the pencil using finger movement. Then try to move it back to the original position.

12. Pencil windmill – hold pencil in the air, with the writing hand, try to turn it like a windmill, using only the hand that is holding the pencil. Try clockwise and anti-clockwise.

13. Hold a pen top, or similar short cylindrical object, between thumb and index and middle fingers and try to turn it round and round clockwise, then anti-clockwise. Then try rolling it down to the base of the thumb/fingers and back up to the top.

14. Right hand then left hand (vice versa if left-handed) press each finger in turn to tip of thumb. Then try both hands together. Eyes open then eyes closed.

15. Put sticky tape on the pad of the index finger, with a bit of tape protruding. Try to get the tape off, using each of the other fingers of the same hand in turn. Repeat with other hand.

16. Place a rubber band over the fingers and the thumb in a loose but just firm fit. Wriggle the fingers and thumb 'open and shut'/together and apart to get the band off. To begin with put the rubber band near the top of the digits then lower down as skill increases. Try different combinations – one finger and thumb, two fingers and thumb, two adjoining fingers…

17. Pressing elbows to sides, point hands and fingers forwards, then one hand at a time rotate hand from wrist, keeping rest of body still.

18. Arm distance from wall, place hands palm down flat to wall and press down on palms and fingers, then use fingers to push back upright. This can be repeated using the table.

19. Place palm flat on table, raise one finger at a time. One hand at a time, then both together.

20. Put hands flat on table, keep fingers straight and move the index finger away from the middle finger, then the index and middle fingers away from the ring finger, then the little finger away from the other fingers. Repeat several times.

21. Hold thumb and next two fingers in cutting/position, as if using scissors, and practise scissor/ cutting movement.

22. Rub hands/fingers briskly.

23. Elbows on table, press heels of hands together, curl fingers, tips apart, then touch corresponding tips one at a time. Eyes open then eyes closed.

24. Sometimes it is helpful to do good sitting, then let chin drop to chest, shoulders droop, close eyes and breathe quietly before starting to write.

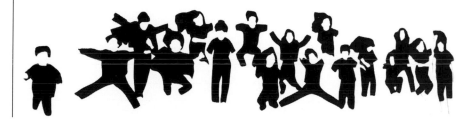

Record chart

Key

J: Jerky, heavy footed, not flowing or controlled
S: Sustains pose or movements for ? seconds
D: Needing demonstration and reminder
W: Wobbly, arms or hands waving or up in hypertensive position, losing balance easily
F: Arms flailing

Name	Date	Date	Date
Good crawling, creeping			
Good standing			
Walks steadily			
Can walk on toes			
Can walk on heels			
Along line/bench			
Up/down steps alternate feet			
Heel to toe			
Standing leg balance			
Standing leg swing			
Stand circle toes in air			
Good balance on knees			
Bridge			
Good sitting			
Good stand from sitting & v v			
Squat balance/bounce			
Rock in swan position bwrds/fwrds			
Curled on back rock side to side			
Sit & spin			
Standing twist			
Cat's got measles			
Shoulder raise singly & both tog			
Shoulder fwrds & bwrds singly & both tog			
Standing scissor arm swing			
Arm rotation			
Straight arm stretch			
Sustained hops			
Sustained jumps			
Skips			
Skips with rope			
Throw, catch, bounce ball			
Finger flex			
Finger curl			
Close fingers smoothly onto palm starting with little finger			
Fingers to thumb, one at time			
Elbows to waist, arms parallel to ground rotate wrists			
Kneeling hands flat on floor rock fwrd weight on wrists			
Cross lateral exercises			
Relax, be still			

5

Curriculum

It will be clear that the speech and language difficulties described so far, will directly affect learning in all areas of the curriculum.

Speech Production

It may be hard to understand what a child is saying when:

- Joining in class or group discussions.
- Answering questions.
- Asking questions.
- Reading his/her own work or other texts.
- Spelling out loud.

It may therefore, be more difficult for a child to show what he or she knows and for the teacher to assess progress.

Vocabulary

Some children will have great difficulty with specific curriculum vocabulary:

- Pronouncing – 'manget' for magnet, 'ecectrility' for electricity.
- Understanding – left can mean gone or remaining, or the opposite to right.
- Remembering.
- Spelling.
- Recognising and using particular words or operational signs, patterns, shapes, place value, the decimal point and numerators/ denominators.

Grammar

Words and word parts may be omitted, letters, words and sentences jumbled when:

- Joining in class or group discussions.
- Answering questions.
- Asking questions.
- Reading aloud.
- Spelling out loud.
- Recording curriculum work.

Listening and Understanding

Some children will have great difficulty in:

- Focusing at the start of a lesson.
- Processing, understanding, remembering all the given information.
- Following instructions during the lesson.

6

Memory

Some children will have great difficulty in trying to remember facts. This can cause panic and overload and result in a total loss of focus on the lesson or task. They may have problems with:

- Sequences of instructions.
- Specific vocabulary and facts.
- Recalling different information, which makes it difficult for them to link subjects across the curriculum area and hinders their problem-solving ability.

Social use of language

Behaviour in class, including class, group and paired discussion and working may be affected as some children will have difficulty in:

- Understanding and remembering different routines or codes within each class, possibly resulting in a difficulty with settling down.
- Relating to others and behaving appropriately with others.
- Remembering and using turn-taking procedures and ways of contributing in class.

Developmental co-ordination

Some children will have great difficulty in:

- Drawing pictures or diagrams, copying from a board, book or workcard.
- Writing words or numbers correctly.
- Handling and using equipment including scissors, pencils, pens, rubbers and rulers and other measuring tools.
- Differentiating between right and left, and so have problems writing on lines right to left and top to bottom on a page.
- Deciding what equipment they need and organising all equipment in their working space so they have enough room to work.
- Appreciating sequential pattern, and sequencing the findings of an investigation.
- Identifying similar words – see/seeds, wet/went...

These are generic problems that all teaching staff need to understand. The following sections cover some subject-specific ideas.

6

English

Speaking and Listening

All the games and activities described in chapters 2 and 3 can be part of speaking and listening work.

Reading

- It is possible for unintelligible children to be reading accurately but to be unable to articulate the words. This is a tricky area but there is no need to hold up reading experience if your instinct indicates that they are reading accurately. Understanding and recall of sight vocabulary can be checked and developed using visual skills – matching, highlighting, pointing to etc.

- Collect and create simple teacher-made books with target vocabulary or grammar in them. We have a set of concept books on wet/dry, hard/soft, colours and some teacher-made books that start at a very early sentence level – Mum is walking, the boy is writing etc. Some children will make a start with simple, personally designed books. Have available as wide a range of books as possible, sorted along Reading Recovery lines, into stages that increase in difficulty in very small steps with lots of repetition.

- The Paget Gorman signing system, which was designed to support the development of spoken language in children with speech and language impairment, actively helps with the learning of a core sight vocabulary. It gives a visual clue and support can be given without interrupting the flow of reading, particularly with words such as '**in, the, is**' and confusions like '**was/went**'.

- Traditional tales and nursery rhymes frequently feature in school readers so it is useful to give these extra attention. Some children may not have heard them much and others may have heard them but do not readily recall them. We regularly take these as our topic theme, and plan a range of curriculum work around it.

- Story tapes – these are available for all ages with or without accompanying books. It can also be of great benefit to some children to use teacher-made tapes that are linked to current class-work.

- It is very important to check understanding, some children can decode well so seem to be reading well but are not reading with understanding. They need lots of practice at answering simple questions (Appendix 4), predicting what will happen next and re-telling the story.

- Some text layouts are more difficult to follow than others, so keep this in mind when selecting suitable reading books.

- Some children will have great difficulty recalling character names, place names and previous events as well as core words. Be ready to

6

support the flow of reading by reminding the child of these words, before he starts to read. During reading, if a given clue does not trigger recall, then tell the child the word to keep the flow of the reading and make the reading session more enjoyable. Then plan for some practice of target names at another time. Acknowledge the child's memory difficulties in a positive way, as outlined earlier. Set realistic targets about teaching techniques for decoding and developing a core sight vocabulary.

● Some children may have difficulties tracking across a page or focusing on words, and for some the words may move around or flicker. If a child appears to be having difficulty or screws up his eyes a lot, or his eyes water a lot when reading, then suggest to parents that they arrange for a sight test. Simple eye exercises can help, and some children have tinted glasses. Try using a tracker, these can be bought from a supplier, or make them out of a rectangle of card with an opening cut in the centre. You can use this to outline a sentence, or two or three sentences, by adjusting the size of the opening. You can also try different colours of cellophane paper to make your own filters.

● Help the children to organise their reading equipment by having a regular routine. Teach them what should be in their book bag or rucksack, and when it should be in school. Reward them when they remember.

Writing

● Use shared contexts or given inputs to start with, to help in understanding exactly what those children with speech production difficulties are saying when they are reading back their work.

● Teach a core written vocabulary.

● Be realistic about how many spellings and how much grammar you expect to be correct, depending on each child's difficulties and targets. Obviously you will have a teaching programme for spelling and grammar in place.

● Use a structured dictionary system.
This may start with a *'Breakthrough to Literacy'* approach, so the children can make sentences with support and read them to a few friends before copying them. Cardboard finger spaces can be used alongside the cardboard words to encourage spaces to be left when copy writing. Move on to using a teacher-made open personal dictionary (Appendix 6). These dictionaries can be used in a number of ways. Children can finger-trace words using a *look, cover, write* method while they are learning a core written vocabulary. They can find their own words and later the initial letter of words. They can begin to try their own spelling.

- Picture sequences can be used at first to retell stories. Tell the story and let the children act it out the day before, or some days before the writing, to develop memory skills. In this way children become confident as they have something to write about and they can build up a repertoire of storylines. When they are confident at this you can try:
  Changing a character, a setting, an event...
  Demonstrating how to storyboard the story with the changes (using blank cartoon type boxes to draw the key events of the story).

- When the children are confident at retelling and changing in this way, move on to story planning with storyboards, using a single picture/event/item as a stimulus. Some children need to be specifically taught how to do quick pictures or else they will spend all the available time drawing. Most children with SLI need support whilst practising how to write their story from a storyboard.

- When the children start to try their own spellings give them a 'Have-a-Go' book. This encourages independent spelling, keeps a record of spelling progression and enables discussion and use of correct spelling.

- As often as possible, encourage the children to talk through what they are going to write a number of times:- before they start, during the writing, and at the finish to check they have kept to their plan. They can also be encouraged to check they have included all words and maybe choose one or two spellings that they have had a good try with but recognise do not look correct.

- Show the children what to do with lots of teacher-led writing demonstrations, using examples that they can then refer to during the writing process.

- Use writing frames for different kinds of writing – letters, poems, informational writing and/or dictionary sheets to support these.

- Read lots of different poetry to the children and show them it doesn't always rhyme. Using cloze is useful, with the children filling in specific words in a given framework. Alternatively, use large strips of paper and during the input write down exactly what each child says, using the kind of prompting outlined earlier in the Expressive Language – Vocabulary section.

- Introduce the children to written recipes during cookery sessions and use a recipe format to write a poem e.g. Autumn – Take a cupful of conkers, a tablespoon of yellow leaves, a tablespoon of red leaves...

- Use ICT: we have recently purchased Clicker 4, which enables personal screens to be set up for each pupil. It is like an on-screen concept keyboard and it is a big plus since it has speech and graphics and can be used for a range of curriculum work.

6

- Older pupils may benefit from portable, tabletop vocabulary reference charts and story-planning charts.

- Give experience of different styles of writing and purposes for writing – thank you letter, postcard etc. and link to social skills being covered. Linking this to role-play with younger children is very useful.

Spelling

In my class rhythm and rhyme work are seen as the first stage of spelling:

Rhythm work. Some activities have been given earlier in the 'Expressive Language – Speech Production' section.

- Tapping out children's names.
- Tapping out a selection of words with different numbers of syllables.
- Tapping out words from current topic vocabulary.
- Tapping different rhythm patterns in music.
- Moving the whole body to different rhythms in folk and modern dance.

As the children become adept at tapping syllables a recording system can be used whereby a counter or pencil mark is put on a grid for each syllable. Later this system can be used to show the number of letters in a word.

Rhyme

Our experience and current research has shown the importance of rhyme.

- Listen to and learn nursery rhymes and other age-appropriate rhymes.

- Play about with well-known rhymes and make up new possibilities e.g.. Humpty Dumpty sat on a chair/rug/dish etc. Humpty Dumpty had curly hair/a new mug/a big fish etc.

- Recite nursery rhymes leaving a space for group to recite the missing rhyming word – Jack and Jill went up the ——.

- Recite nursery rhymes but put in the wrong word and children have to stand up if they hear a wrong word, then tell you what it was – Jack and Jill went up the stairs etc.

- Reverse words – Song a sing of sixpence/Jill and Jack went up the hill.

- Substitute words – Baa baa purple sheep/Twinkle, twinkle little car.

- Swap word order – Humpty Dumpty wall on a sat/Jack fell down and crown his broke.

- Swap word parts – 1,2 shuckle my boo/I'm a little teapot, shawl and tout/Incy wincy spider went up the spater wout.

- Rhyming pairs or snap. Identify and chant the rhymes together first, then take turns round the circle to pick up 2 cards at a time looking for the pairs. Or give 1 card to each child (making sure there are pairs of rhyming words) the first child stands and says his/her word e.g. '*hat*' and the child with the rhyming card stands and says his/her rhyme then all chant the rhyme.

- Use rhyming picture cards. Lay them out face up. Start the game by saying 'I need a word that rhymes with *hat*', the children look for rhyming cards (have more than one if possible) and put hands up to identify. You could have counters and award a counter for each one found.

- 'My basket is full of **cheese**.' Say the line then throw a beanbag to friend who says it again but gives a different rhyme (peas, fleas, trees, bees, keys, or any nonsense rhyme – mees, rees…)
  Other starter lines:
  My basket is full of logs
  My basket is full of hats
  My basket is full of cars etc…

- Rhyming I spy. I spy something that rhymes with *ball*.

- Give a rhyme – Ask the children as a group or in turn to fill in the rhyme.

On a log I saw a _____	The boy is tall he can catch the _____
I like to eat a slice of _____	Tears in my eye I started to _____
The pig wore a _____	My sock is on the _____
The star is in the _____	I saw a rat chasing a _____
When we go for a walk I like to _____	The rich king wore a sparkling _____
A fox in a _____	A green snake eating _____
Do you see the little _____	On a dark night the moon shines _____
I saw a mole come out of a _____	6,7,8 shut the _____
The little hen swallowed a _____	Stop singing that song it's much too ____
In a house a little _____	In the sun he had some _____

6

Slightly harder, extended listening and processing.

It is dark, switch on the light.
The sun has set now it's _____

You live in me. I sound like mouse.
I have a roof and walls. I am a _____

You look at me to tell the time.
I rhyme with rock I am a _____

I swim in the river, I sound like dish.
I am a _____

You sit on me I sound like hair.
I am a _____

This is a word that rhymes with make.
It's delicious to eat it is a _____

This is a word that rhymes with jar.
It needs petrol, it is a _____

This is a word that rhymes with king.
It ties things up, it's a ball of _____

This is a word that rhymes with sighs.
You see with these, they are your _____

This is a word that rhymes with run.
Round and sticky it is a _____

This is a word that rhymes with coat.
It sails on the sea it is a _____

This is a word that rhymes with smelly.
It wobbles and wobbles it's delicious ____

Slightly harder, extended listening and processing and thinking.

I'm thinking of something you wear on your feet it rhymes with choose.

I'm thinking of something you wear on your legs it rhymes with lights.

I'm thinking of something you wear when it's cold it rhymes with moat.

I'm thinking of something you wear on your head it rhymes with mat.

I'm thinking of something you wear round your neck it rhymes with laugh.

I'm thinking of something you wear next to your skin it rhymes with best.

I'm thinking of something you wear on your feet it rhymes with candles.

I'm thinking of something boys wear to swim they rhyme with monks.

I'm thinking of something you tuck in your trousers it rhymes with dirt.

After that, or alongside that, a system that teaches letter names, a range of common letter sounds and both upper and lower case has been successful. This emphasises that most letters have more than one common sound. This has been found particularly important with children who have difficulty understanding language and who interpret literally. If they learn that /a/ says a as in apple they will have difficulty accepting it makes other sounds. It is easier to use 'apple begins with **a**', 'apron begins with **a (ay)**' and to mention that the letter a makes many other sounds as well. To this end we start with a wider group of letter/sound combinations and go on to an even wider set later. Jolly Phonics, a system with visual cues, has also proved most helpful but we have adapted it to include extra actions to go with the additional letter sounds as described above.

6

There are many spelling systems about; *Alpha to Omega* by Bevé Hornsby has proved a useful reference. Older pupils have successfully used a package called *Toe by Toe* by Keda Cowling and a computer based *Integrated Learning System*. The *Integrated Learning System* allows regular, structured practise of basic skills in a fun and supportive way.

- Use multi-sensory techniques whereby letters are looked at, finger traced, traced on a range of rough and smooth surfaces, traced with eyes open and closed.
- Link speech articulation work with spelling.
- Use phonological awareness tasks.
- Count the syllables in a word.
- Count the letters/sounds in a word.
- Subtract a syllable e.g. farmyard without farm or into without in.
- Change the first letter but keep the rhyme/word family – cat to hat/rat/sat...
- Link handwriting and spelling. A cursive style from the start has been shown to be really helpful. However, I have found that it is necessary at Key Stage 1 to point out the difference between the way we write the letters and the ways we read them. We have adapted our alphabet reference cards and our core word reference cards to show cursive and non-cursive and we say "This is the way we read it; this is the way we write it."
- Use grids, at first with the correct number of boxes, for spelling particular words.
- Use a range of different letters – plastic, magnetic, foam, cardboard.
- Use teacher-made spellers with cardboard letters attached to a base alphabet by sticky-backed Velcro. We sing the alphabet names, sing a vowel song, practise the common initial sounds of the letters as above and pull off the letters to spell words, chanting the names then the sounds, then the whole word.

cat – see (C) ay (A) tee (T) – /c/ /a/ /t/   cat

The nature of speech and language impairment changes over time and some children with early speech production problems, along with children with other language impairment, go on to have more significant literacy difficulties, sometimes called SpLD (Specific Learning Difficulties) or Dyslexia. Whatever it is called, these children will need specific help with literacy for a considerable time, maybe for all of their schooling.

6

Mathematics

The language of maths

For many children, the actual numerical or spatial work involved in the curriculum is obscured by the language surrounding it. It is therefore essential to spend time on the explicit teaching of mathematical vocabulary and explaining the multiple meanings of the most common words. Plan time for overlearning of vocabulary, in language and in therapy sessions as well as in the numeracy hour.

- If a child is having difficulty consider the language being used, try phrasing it another way and then note the particular maths terms causing difficulty so these can be worked on later. Allow these pupils more time, or let them use concrete materials and visual aids for longer. Also consider whether the maths task has meaning for the child or whether it is too abstract; try to give real examples or at least use concrete materials.
- Use correct and consistent maths terminology, discussing this with pupils. Consider using one term only until a pupil is secure in that process, e.g. use **add** exclusively at first without using **more/plus**, etc.
- Try to include short regular practice of maths vocabulary and procedures. For example, use register time for each child and each member of staff to place their own bottle top under a packed lunch or dinner sign. The bottle tops represent the people present; the idea of representation is an abstract one and it is helpful to practise it like this. We count how many, how many more and less/fewer; we look for the double number. We chant the double numbers from double one up to double ten and, as the year progresses, we chant a range of terms associated with addition and subtraction.

Packed lunch	Dinner
1	1
1	1
1	
1	

This would be 4 packed lunches, 2 dinners, 6 meals altogether.

The double number is 2 with 2 more packed lunches and 2 less (fewer) dinners.

Using fingers we would all show double 2 is 4, 2+2=4, 2 plus 2 is 4, 2 more than 2 is 4, the total of 2 and 2 is 4, 2 count on 2 is 4, 2 and 2 how many altogether?
and
Half of 4 is 2, 4-2=2, 2 less than 4 is 2, 4 count back 2 is 2, the difference between 2 and 4 is 2, subtract 2 from 4 the answer is 2.

In this way the children become familiar with the range of terms and, although they are simply chanting at first, they are taking the first steps towards understanding them.

Volume = level of noise or amount of space taken up or particular book in a series

Left = someone has gone or remaining or the opposite of right

Place = where you are or place value or 'to put'

Change = change (replace) your clothes or change in money (loose coins) or change this number (alter)

6

- It may be helpful to break down AT 1 to include vocabulary and concepts necessary for investigative maths.

	Level 1	Level 2
Making decisions to solve problems	Use maths for practical tasks. Has used a range of maths materials that has been given.	Select/use materials for maths tasks. Selects maths materials for own use.
	Shows interest/involvement in 'finding out'. Talks about practical tasks.	Has experienced different ways of tackling a task. Offers ideas for tackling a task.
Developing mathematical language	Is working hard to learn/ understand a range of maths language. Needs consistent terminology.	Can show understanding of a range of maths language. Uses and relates numerals/ maths symbols/maths language in a range of situations.
	Answers closed questions… Is it full or empty? Is it a circle or a square?	Answers closed questions with a choice of objects… Which is longer? Which is heaviest?
	Completes statements… It isn't full, it's _____ It isn't heavy, it's _____	Answers more open questions. How much/many? What shape/size?
	Makes statements… It's full. This is a circle.	Responds using maths language to "Tell me about this". Asks maths questions.
	Follows simple maths instructions.	Chooses how to record from a given range.
Reasoning	Can continue simple sequences.	Can continue patterns.
	Can make patterns and simply describe them.	Can make patterns and describe them. Can use simple patterns in finding solutions.
	Makes simple predictions by answering appropriately, based on own experience of patterns/ relationships. Do you think this will fit there? Will this balance?	Can appropriately answer 'What would happen if?/Why?' questions. If I put this on the scales it will _____ If I pour this in here it will _____

- In literacy time practise reading for meaning with maths problems and encourage the pupils to expect the text to make sense. Teach the vocabulary involved. Discuss which are the key words/parts of the problem and what the pupil has to do, highlighting the important parts. Use concrete apparatus if needed. When finished, help the pupil to talk through what they did.
- Some children may be easily overwhelmed by the enormity of mental maths and problem-solving tasks and will need help to get started. They may have difficulty with 'why' and 'how' questions and need lots of demonstration and practice in working out what to do to tackle a problem, what operation to use, thinking logically

6

and drawing helpful diagrams. Help pupils clarify their thinking, and select the correct format for recording ideas and solutions.

- Separate number work from more investigative and practical maths, as the language content of these will require particular attention. This affects the way commercially produced materials are used.
- Consider layout carefully, sometimes this can be most confusing: 15-8, 20-4, 8-7 all proceed left to right but 'take 8 away from 10' does not.
- Pay particular attention to maths terms that may be easily confused, e.g. thirteen/thirty, fourteen/forty, and so on.
- Be ready to provide concrete aids for a considerable time and aim for a multi-sensory teaching/learning style. Use sandpaper or textured number reference charts. Have visual aids (tables, charts, diagrams, calculators) available to prompt the memory or to be used if a pupil just can't remember. Make sure that all equipment matches the age and interest level of the pupils and give it all an acceptable status within class. Try to have several or at least more than one aid and have them available for all to use.
- Use class charts to show a range of maths terms such as add, subtract, multiply, divide and equals or use symbols. Each time a new term is encountered it can be added to the chart. (See opposite.)
- Check understanding of left and right and of moving from left to right across the page. Mark right and left on the page; have a right and left reference chart available or put a temporary mark on a pupil's hand. Or show pupils that their left hand makes a capital L when you put it on the table or put a wristband on their right hand.
- Consider the use of some number shortcuts, and actively encourage pupils to give approximate answers against which their eventual answer can be checked.
- Demonstrate and talk through how you reached an answer and ask pupils to talk you through how they have reached an answer. This can show difficulties and some interesting methods you may not be aware of. Obviously, some children will find this really difficult and that in itself reminds you of the difficulties they have in sequential and logical thinking.
- Some mistakes will be due to memory problems or wordfinding difficulties. Accept this and respond sympathetically.
- Check written work frequently so that mistakes can be dealt with early on and, if possible, before the incorrect methods/answers become ingrained and therefore will be remembered as correct. And check work early on in a lesson to ensure correct layout and so there isn't too much re-writing or re-drawing if incorrect.
- Some pupils will benefit from compiling and using a personal reminder book, which has examples of ways of working a problem and particular maths vocabulary with a personal explanation/pictogram.
- Check homework tasks are set out correctly and clearly. Provide ready-prepared sheets where possible rather than expect children to copy from the board.
- Mark the starting point on each page – green for go and the stopping point – red for stop. Use arrows, dotted lines or colours

Use class charts to show a range of maths terms

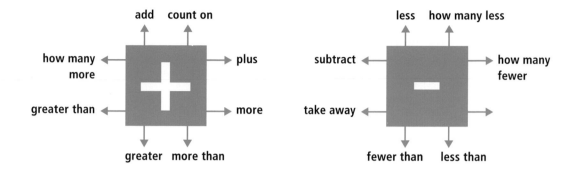

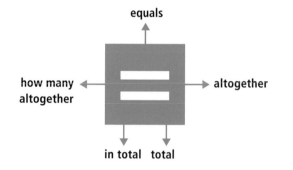

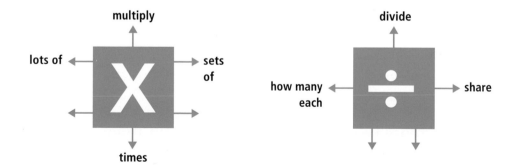

6

to show the way to go across or down the page.

- Teach the writing of numerals in groups where numerals that are being confused are not taught at the same time. If particular numerals are being confused, give each one a different identifying attribute – colour or cartoon/picture.
- Allow the use of number stamps, plastic and stick-on numbers whilst pupils are becoming competent in writing numbers.
- Use different colours for numbers/signs that are confused or place on different coloured card as reference sheets. Or use full arrow shapes for the more and less signs.
- Teach how to use squared paper but continue to use start/stop marker and guides lines, HTU etc.
- Plan for more pattern work, patterns of numbers that make 10, that make 20, within a 100 square, within tables etc.
- Practise the days of the week, months etc as regularly as possible.
- Teach and practise rounding up/down to the nearest ten, so that estimating is easier.
- Encourage children to work in pencil, as it's easier to rub out and redo. Establish the use of rulers for any lines and give time to practise the correct use of a ruler and other drawing and measuring tools. Purchase rulers with handles to help those with co-ordination difficulties.

Many pupils feel anxious about maths and their fears can lead to avoidance strategies like doing work very slowly or disruptive behaviour or even truancy.

- Acknowledge to the pupil that you understand that he or she has to work hard at maths and praise the effort he/she is making.
- Plan for success. Balance set tasks to include a mix of those that pupils can succeed with, and those where support is needed. Have help (visual aids, charts as well as teacher help) organised and available when it is needed.
- Be aware of each pupil's coping strategies and explain these to helpers and parents.
- Avoid asking anxious pupils to answer aloud at first and establish a supportive environment wherein any contribution is welcomed and praised and 'good thinking' is highlighted and discussed.
- Create opportunities for collaborative working.

Each pupil with SLI will present with a different pattern of difficulties and abilities and it is likely that each will have a mix of problems. It will be necessary to establish priorities for each pupil to ensure overlearning and re-visiting of vital pre-number and early maths knowledge. Some children with speech and language impairment have an aptitude for maths computation and experience their first feelings of success with number work, but need particular help with the language of maths. Others find all maths work extremely difficult and need lots of praise for their courage and the enormous effort they make in tackling it rather than for the end result.

Science

Problem-solving, knowledge of facts and understanding specific terminology are areas that are central to Science as well as Maths. Some children will have difficulty pronouncing Science terminology. This in turn will affect their recall, understanding and use of some words. Try to include short regular practice of some vocabulary and use class charts/wall displays to show a range of terms.

Much of the vocabulary and language concepts that underpin science are covered on the First Words list (Appendix 2). It is useful to target specific vocabulary in language sessions as well as science sessions and also to involve parents where possible, in using opportunities to practise the words at home, e.g. (same/different, changed/change/change back, longer/shorter, wider/narrower, rougher/smoother...)

- If a child is having difficulty in understanding the language being used, try phrasing it another way and then note the particular science terms causing difficulty so these can be worked on later. Also consider whether the science task has meaning for the child or whether it is too abstract; try to give real examples or use concrete materials.
- Plan for regular, short sessions practising vocabulary and use chanting, singing, or actions to aid learning and remembering.
- Provide illustrated science dictionary sheets for class use.
- Provide and encourage the use of reference charts, diagrams and concrete materials and give them an acceptable status by making them available for all to use.
- Use pupil reminder books where examples of particular science vocabulary with a personal explanation/pictogram are noted.
- Aim for a multi-sensory teaching/learning style.
- Remember there may be difficulties with understanding verbal explanations and instructions and this may affect investigation work. Pupils may need lots of demonstration and supervised practice in working out what to do to tackle an investigation.
- Demonstrate and talk through how a decision has been reached.
- Provide frameworks for recording activities and findings.
- In literacy time practise reading for meaning with science investigations and encourage the pupils to expect the text to make sense. Teach the vocabulary involved, discuss which are the key words/parts of the problem and what the pupil has to do, and highlight the important parts. Use concrete apparatus if needed. When finished, help the pupil to talk through what they did.
- Some children will have particular difficulties with AT 1 where they are expected to hypothesise. We have found it helpful to break down the targets for AT 1 as detailed over.
- Check written work frequently so that errors can be dealt with before they become learnt as correct and while the pupil remembers the task. Provide frameworks for recording and use a variety of methods – highlighting, circling, matching, cutting and pasting given pictures.

6

Experimental and Investigative

1	Beginning to recognise same and different.	Is interested, chooses to observe materials, displays.	Given a reminder, uses senses when observing.	Can answer closed questions. (Is it hot?) (Can it bend?)
	Can answer forced alternatives. (Is it rough or smooth?)	Can complete statements. (It isn't hard it's _____)	With help joins in simple discussion. Beginning to offer own ideas.	Draws simple charts to communicate ideas.
2	Chooses from given ideas of how an investigation should proceed.	Answers one option questions. (Will this sink if I put it in the water?)	Answers How and What questions. (How does it move? What is it made of?)	Listens and selects likely ideas from given ones of "What might happen if".
	Makes observations.	With some help uses own ideas.	Has used a range of simple equipment.	Records findings. Can say if they were expected.
3	Responds to suggestions of how to create an investigation.	Makes own suggestions of how to create an investigation.	Asks relevant questions. (How/Why/what will happen if?)	Makes predictions.
	Makes relevant observations. Uses a range of equipment, takes measurements.	With help will carry out fair test. Knows and can explain why it is fair.	Records in a variety of ways.	Can explain observations and any patterns found in measurements. Can say what they have found out from work.

- Allow adequate time for neat work and if necessary build in practice time, practising writing / drawing faster whilst maintaining neatness. Link this to investigative work – set up a fair test on adequate time for recording work.

In Science, teachers can directly target vocabulary and concept work and build in lots of 'hands on' experiences so that children with speech and language impairment can thoroughly enjoy the subject. Pupils will steadily become more confident with science vocabulary and straightforward knowledge, though they often need support with making sensible predictions and in generalising their findings. It is necessary then to establish priorities for each pupil to ensure appropriate 're-visiting' and consolidation of knowledge and skills.

6

Wider Curriculum

As previously stated the general difficulties given at the start of this section apply to all areas of the curriculum. It is worth giving further thought to vocabulary since when the whole curriculum is taken into consideration there is a wealth of vocabulary to be learned. It is essential to be realistic and set each child achievable aims as far as the amount of vocabulary to be covered and, hopefully, remembered.

In History and Geography the following is the vocabulary we target. However, we are aware that for some of our children this will not be consistently remembered or understood by the end of Key Stage 1.

History

Chronological awareness:

Can sequence a set of picture cards into a logical order. 2/ 3/ 4/ 5/ 6/ more			Can sequence a set of picture cards and give a spoken description or account of the event. 2/ 3/ 4/ 5/ 6/ more		
Can sequence and show understanding of:			Can show understanding and recall vocabulary for use:		
Yesterday	Today	Tomorrow	Today/ Yesterday/ Tomorrow	Days of the week	Months/ A year/ Years old/ Age
What I have already done	What I am doing	What I'm going to do next	Seasons	Night/ Day	Morning/ afternoon/ evening
This morning	This afternoon	This evening	Old/ new	Old/ young	Clock times
When I was a baby	Now	When I grow up	Before/ after/ afterwards	Soon/ now/ later/ then	Once/ Often/ Usually
Old	New		Suddenly	Again	Sometimes/ Never
When Gran was little	When Mum was little	Now I'm little	While/ Yet/ Until	Already/ Always	Almost/ Nearly
Long, long ago	Long ago	Now	Real/ imaginary	Alive/ dead	Adult, grown-up/ child

Geography

Shows understanding and can recall for use:

In/ on/ under/ behind/ in front/ up/ down/ over/ off/ out/ top/ bottom/ next to/ between/ against/ far/ near/ high/ low/ corner/ middle/ edge/ big/ little/ long/ short/ tall/ short/ wide/ narrow/ thick/ thin/ deep/ shallow/ above/ below/ along/ forwards/ backwards/ sideways/ across/ through/ back/ front/ at/ to/ from/ about/ beside/ into/ out of/ together/ apart/ around/ towards/ away from/ inside/ outside/ anywhere/ everywhere/ nowhere/ somewhere/ here/ where/ there.
Vocabulary connected with vehicles/ weather/ buildings/ jobs/ town and country

In Art, Design, ICT, PE and Music we focus on providing as much enjoyable 'hands on' experience as possible. The vocabulary we have prioritised in these subjects is included in our First Words list (Appendix 2). In this way overlearning is built in as this vocabulary is addressed in language work as well as specific curriculum tasks. This vocabulary has been carefully chosen but not designated to particular curriculum subjects since there are so many overlaps e.g. position words could go under Language, Maths, PE, Geography, Music, Art, Design or ICT.

Some children with speech and language impairment have considerable success learning a second language but it has to be accepted that some find it very difficult. In Wrexham our children learn Welsh as a second language and it is my experience that many of them find it very difficult. So we limit the vocabulary and use it repeatedly with visual aids, role-play, songs and rhymes.

General points

- Questioning is used in all curriculum areas and it may be helpful to consider the nature of questions and their hierarchy of complexity (Appendix 4). The Guess Who game is particularly useful for developing questioning skills.
- In addition to considering the methods and the language content of teaching and instruction it may be useful to consider the structure of a lesson or input. The NFER (National Federation for Educational Research) has carried out some research into the structure of effective lessons. A style they found to be effective for all pupils, including those with some special educational need, is given opposite.

This is a familiar way of working for many colleagues and it is good to have it officially acknowledged as constructive.

When considering the development of language, as mentioned above, play and 'hands on' activities are essential. Play situations can be set up to teach particular vocabulary or language concepts. Play can be structured to reinforce or overlearn this language, then later the children will, hopefully, incorporate the same language in their own play.

Play can give an opportunity to relate language to something concrete; something that can be touched, seen, smelt, and tasted, something that can be directly experienced. This ensures that language is used meaningfully, which is especially important for our children.

Play can lead to the exploration and development of particular manipulative skills, organisational skills, imagination and reading and writing skills. For instance, dressing and undressing the dolls helps the children develop their own dressing skills whilst role-play can develop a depth of understanding in topic work and allows for reading and writing with a purpose.

In specialist settings the children work intensively. Usually there is an adult on hand expecting a 'best try' and unless we plan carefully there is little 'down time'. 'Down time' is needed for the children to relax, to unwind a little and to recharge their batteries. The bonus is that

6

Structure for effective lessons

● A short introduction when:

the purpose of the lesson is given

the main points from the previous lesson are
reviewed

specific vocabulary is introduced

the main information that is to be presented is
identified

● Time to explore materials/resources.

● Instructional period of information giving.
For older pupils it is helpful to provide a written
outline so that the pupil can concentrate on the
presentation rather than on taking notes. An
alternative is to pair the pupils so that one pupil
who takes notes easily can accurately take notes
that can be photocopied later for the other pupil.

● Task setting followed by paired or small group work.

● Verbal summary of findings in groups then report
back to class as a whole.
It is very helpful for pupils to talk through what
they have learned, it gives an indication of how
well they have understood the work.

● Recording of findings to an agreed format which
may include a cloze exercise or words and
pictograms.

6

during these times, through play and activities, they can be consolidating language work already covered in a more intense session.

Difficulties with language may have meant that some children were unable to derive much benefit or enjoyment from play; they may have missed out on some of the ordinary, day-to-day experiences and social development that occurs through play in the early years at home. Many of our young children with speech and language impairment have not participated in much play at all. As their language skills develop they need the opportunity to experience successful play situations they may have missed in earlier years.

Successful play encourages language development, and language and communication are an integral part of successful play.

6

Parents as Part of the Team

Developing effective parent professional working is beneficial for all those involved.

But like everything else it requires careful thought and planning. To establish effective parent professional partnerships it is necessary:

- To establish a climate wherein contributions from either party are valued and respected.
- For professionals to increase their knowledge and understanding of the parent perspective and check that parents have a clear idea of the school's expectations.
- To develop good communication and counselling skills.

The three quotes below illustrate the experiences of some parents of children with speech and language impairment and highlight some points for consideration.

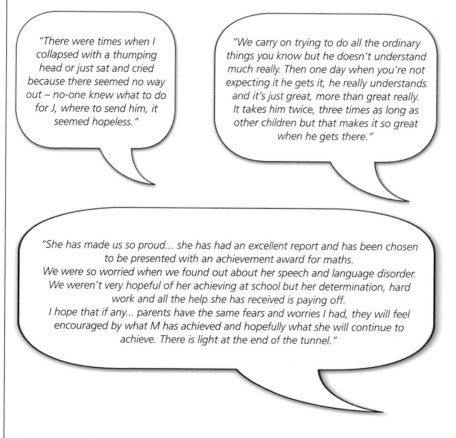

"There were times when I collapsed with a thumping head or just sat and cried because there seemed no way out – no-one knew what to do for J, where to send him, it seemed hopeless."

"We carry on trying to do all the ordinary things you know but he doesn't understand much really. Then one day when you're not expecting it he gets it, he really understands and it's just great, more than great really. It takes him twice, three times as long as other children but that makes it so great when he gets there."

"She has made us so proud... she has had an excellent report and has been chosen to be presented with an achievement award for maths.
We were so worried when we found out about her speech and language disorder. We weren't very hopeful of her achieving at school but her determination, hard work and all the help she has received is paying off.
I hope that if any... parents have the same fears and worries I had, they will feel encouraged by what M has achieved and hopefully what she will continue to achieve. There is light at the end of the tunnel."

Parents may have a frustrating time trying to get their child's difficulties recognised and then a struggle trying to secure an appropriate placement or appropriate support. Be aware when first meeting parents of children with speech and language difficulties, that the stressful time they have had may affect the way they approach you.

- Plan for a smooth and happy start in school to reassure pupil and parents.
- Establish a good system of communication with parents. Even if the school already has a system in place, consider whether it meets the needs of parents of pupils with special needs, including those with speech and language impairment. Such parents will benefit from more frequent meetings and exchanges of information. It is beneficial for parents and professionals to work together on any individual targets and regular liaison is needed for this too. Some schools use a daily diary system, others use the reading diary that goes home regularly whilst others prefer to talk at the end of each day. Whatever system is chosen it needs to be one that suits both school and parents.
- Consider a system for emergencies. Some children with speech and language impairment will not show any anxiety or unhappiness at school but will wait until they get home. Parents are then left in a frustrating and unhappy position, with a distraught child who may not sleep that night and will probably refuse to go to school the next day.
- Consider potentially difficult times – both inside and outside the classroom situation (speech therapy, special needs sessions, transition from one key stage to another, from mainstream to specialist provision or from specialist provision to mainstream).
- Raise awareness, amongst all staff and volunteer helpers, of speech and language difficulties and effective ways of helping children.
- Be aware of the strain that parents may be under. Living with a children with language difficulties can prove exhausting.
- Continue to be sensitive as to how any messages or information about progress or lack of it, may be received. Parents may experience a wide range of emotions from anger, through despair to hope.
- Having considered how best to support pupils with speech and language impairment in your educational setting, try to implement strategies as whole-class or whole-school strategies. Whole-school listening and playground strategies can benefit not just the children with speech and language impairment, but all children in school.
- Be very clear to parents about whole-school and whole-class strategies and support, as well as any individual support their child will be receiving.
- Find out about local and national support agencies and information centres, and help parents to decipher the educational jargon in official documents (see Appendix 9).

Reviews

Whether through a review of the child's statement of special educational need, or the school's own monitoring system, more formal meetings will need to take place at least once a year. These meetings need careful planning so they can be as relaxed, informative and useful as possible.

- Give enough time and information in advance so that each person

'For parents of children with special needs there is often no clear path, expectations and assumptions have to be constantly revised, there is shock, bewilderment, isolation and sadness and anger and at the same time there is often pressure (self-imposed or from outside) to take action, to make decisions and to 'deal with' the situation'.

Blamires M et al. Parent Teacher Partnership (1997) David Fulton

'For parents almost any meeting about their child feels like a crisis meeting'

(Blamires et al 1997)

attending can contribute. Consider giving a brief framework of the areas to be discussed so questions and points can be thought through, jotted down and brought to the meeting. Parents may welcome some help in compiling their own contribution. If this is established procedure for parents and professionals then such points can be discussed in a non-threatening way.

- Offer parents the opportunity to bring a friend so they don't feel quite so outnumbered by professionals.
- Consider the environment in which the meeting will be held. It needs to be a place where the meeting can proceed without interruption. The furniture needs to be arranged so the room is welcoming and relaxed.
- Appoint a facilitator and a scribe. The facilitator should invite each person present to speak and ensure there is time for everyone to make a contribution. The facilitator should also feed back regularly throughout the meeting, what has been discussed and decided and at the close of the meeting summarise the main points and decisions. The scribe should keep an eye on the time and be responsible for taking minutes which will be distributed to all those present as soon as possible after the meeting.
- All those present need to be introduced or to introduce themselves.
- Check your body language to ensure it is welcoming and attentive.
- Guard against giving an honest but totally negative report.
- Engage in active listening – show that you really want to hear what others have to say, respect their feelings and opinions even if they differ from your own.
- Try not to take expressions of strong feelings, rage or sadness personally.
- Deal with any friction or distress sensitively, ask questions to elicit more information e.g. "Can you tell us why this is annoying/ upsetting you?"
- Allow everyone to make final comments and set a date for the next meeting.

These may seem to be very basic points but I have found that a checklist based on the points above ensures meetings are friendly and useful.

Working together

Be ready to work with parents but be wary of over burdening them. Sarah Newman (*Small Steps Forward*, 1999 Jessica Kingsley) wrote:

'All the specialists bombard you with leaflets and things to do and you feel you should be doing everything all at once or that you are never doing enough and sometimes your child is unresponsive or unco-operative and you feel overwhelmed and an abject failure'.

Accept that for some parents, just surviving the ordinary daily routine is all they can manage, whilst for others, just doing ordinary family things is worthwhile and more than enough. Such parents may not be able to become so involved for a variety of reasons ranging from lack of confidence to work commitments. They may need more direct

"I'll tell you what it's like sometimes. He doesn't understand and stamps and screams in a rage. His grandparents and my sister criticise me for not disciplining him, they don't understand and think I should be firm with him. He's upset, I'm upset and in the middle his brother wants help with his homework. It's exhausting."

support and it may require more time and effort to establish and maintain good communication. Many parents may still be coming to terms with their child's impairment and will need sensitivity and understanding. (Garry Hornby compares this to the grieving process. His thoughts on this are very helpful in gaining some understanding of the feelings of parents of children with special needs.)

Other parents will be, or will become, very knowledgeable about speech and language impairment and will wish to be very involved in supporting their child. They will be active members of the team, probably coming into school to work alongside staff, if this is your policy. When this type of arrangement is established, it can be beneficial for all, especially the child concerned.

Children with speech and language difficulties need opportunities to practise their developing speech and language skills. They need opportunities to experience a range of language concepts and vocabulary at first hand. They may need to improve their co-ordination skills. Parents and other family members can help with all of these. In fact, by providing opportunities in their home environments they are providing different contexts and helping their child both to generalise and to consolidate learning. Some things are done better at home – there are banks of vocabulary that are much more meaningful when experienced outside school – animals, vehicles etc. It is easier to have extended conversations at home and to have the undivided attention of a person or small group of people.

Parents and professionals working together can help their children learn in a more complete and holistic way, and often at a faster pace. Certainly, and perhaps most importantly of all, when partnership working is successful and a child makes progress, the sense of achievement and joy is felt by all those involved – pupil, parent and professional.

'I was at the end of my tether when T eventually got some support, exhausted and drained. I wanted him to get help but I wanted him to not need it, to be in an ordinary class. So I was down too, a bit depressed. I thought it was all my fault. Then things began to change. The first thing was he was happier, he loved going to school. And then I started to come in and watch you, what you did and I'd tell you what he'd done at home and you'd tell me about school, good and bad so we could work together. It was easier, I didn't get so fraught because we helped each other. Now he's making progress with some things but not much with others, like maths. But he's getting the help he needs and we've started to feel hopeful about the future.'

Concluding Thoughts

Children with Speech and language impairment may present with a range of difficulties affecting all areas of the curriculum and they may be viewed as having significant special educational needs.

Conversely, if approached another way, all curriculum areas can be used to support the development of language skills and learning in general by acknowledging that some children learn differently. Then it is a short step to planning for this different learning:

- **Speech production** – Clear, flowing speech, conversation skills and question and answer techniques can be practised as part of group and class discussions within a supportive environment wherein any contribution is welcomed and praised and 'good thinking' is highlighted, demonstrated and discussed.
- **Vocabulary** – Vocabulary can be prioritised within each curriculum subject, flagged up at the start of the session, briefly recapped during and at the end of a session, and used during follow-up work.
- **Grammar** – Grammar is an important part of literacy work but can also be part of developing recording skills in other curriculum areas, directly taught.
- **Listening skills** – A whole-school approach works best: short introductory inputs, reminders and praise for specific listening behaviours (good sitting, good looking, good thinking, turn-taking).
- **Understanding** – Check understanding regularly in a variety of different ways, throughout every lesson.
- **Memory skills** – These are part of listening and understanding as pupils are called upon to remember the vocabulary and knowledge content of a session. Short revision times can be built into any lesson, with pupils using supportive aids if appropriate.
- **Social use of language techniques** – These are part of good listening and part of a whole-school behaviour and discipline policy. In addition they can be addressed during PSHE and RE sessions.
- **Acceptable behaviour** – This too is part of a whole-school behaviour and discipline policy. Teaching acceptable behaviours can be carried out in context during the school day - e.g. quieter voices in class/louder in PE, or how to organise sharing equipment, acceptable ways forward, who to go to and how to ask for help when a task seems impossible.
- **Co-ordination** – Specific extra daily sessions to develop motor skills are relatively easy to build into the school day. Short warm-up sessions, for whole-body movement or manipulative skills can be built in at lining-up times as well as at the beginning of lessons – PE or writing, art, design or cookery.
- **Sensory integration** – Short tasks or routines to develop sensory integration can be built into daily class routines – such as a feelings board, movement breaks, posture cushions and legitimate 'fiddle toys' alongside the use of multi-sensory techniques.

In our busy, over-full school days anything that takes extra time at the planning stage may initially seem to be unhelpful. However, the population of children with speech and language difficulties is significant, and some of these children will remain in mainstream classes for most, if not all, of their education. There is a need then for colleagues, in both specialist and mainstream settings, to increase their knowledge of speech and language difficulties and how best to support these children. It would be helpful if many of the suggestions that have been given become part of general good practice so that all children, those with particular special needs and those without, will benefit. All pupils benefit from clear and straightforward instructional language and from clear target-setting based on individual needs. So in the long term time is saved, as teaching becomes more effective for all pupils.

Speech and language impairment is a relatively new field of study and as such we are learning more about it all the time. The ideas given in this book are offered in a spirit of collaborative working and it is hoped that, as practitioners in the classroom situation, colleagues in mainstream will work with specialist teachers to improve on current practice and make school an enjoyable and successful experience for all children.

> **Mrs M:** *Why do we come to school?*
>
> **C:** *I know, I know it's… we learn… we learn… we learn **everything**.*
>
> **Mrs M:** *Okay, and why do you think it's important to learn at school?*
>
> **C:** *Good thinking , we learn good thinking… cos when we are growned ups… it will… it will be a good earth and we can have a **good time**.*

Stages of Language Development

The developmental stages outlined below have been taken from a number of sources, including Sheridan and Crystal. They can only ever be a very rough guide, and care should be taken, particularly when working with parents, to ensure an understanding of the wide variation in patterns of 'normal' development.

Expressive Language

1-9 months

- **1 month** – startled by loud noises, stiffens, blinks and may cry. At first all cries are pure reflex but by 6 weeks there are different cries for hunger, discomfort, etc. This is the beginning of communication. There may be reflex babbling.
- By **3 months** – there is a definite response to mother's voice, vocalisation when spoken to, may turn towards sound.
- By **6 months** – turns immediately to mother's voice across a room, vocalises tunefully with single and double sounds, lots of babbling, intonation patterns emerging and often recognisable.

9-18 months

- **9–12 months** – vocalises deliberately, shouts to attract attention, listens and shouts again. Babbles tunefully, echoes sounds and simplified words with no understanding, some imitation of adult sounds. Responds to own name and understands 'no' and 'bye - bye' and accompanying gestures.
- By **12 months** – shows understanding of several words in context, familiar names such as 'dinner', 'car', etc. Comprehends simple commands given with gestures – 'Give it to daddy', 'Clap hands'. Uses one or two words with understanding.
- By **15 months** – spoken vocabulary of between 6-10 words, mostly nouns, verbs and other words such as 'more', 'there', 'all', 'gone', 'yes', 'no', familiar names and some question words like 'what', 'where', 'who'. Jabbers loudly and freely, using a wide range of inflection and phonetic units, experiments with sounds. Vocalises wishes and needs, points to familiar persons, animals or toys when requested. Understands many more than 6-10 words and obeys simple commands such as 'Shut the door', 'Give me the ball'.

18 months-2 years

- A spoken vocabulary of 6-20 words and understands many more. Uses jargon and much gesture. Often echoes last word of what is said to him. Demands desired objects by pointing and loud, urgent vocalisation of single words. Tries to sing, enjoys nursery rhymes and tries to join in.
- By **2 years** – more verbal expression, less jargon. Uses 50 or more words and understands many more. May begin to join words to make simple sentences. A vocabulary of around 50 words is needed before two words are meaningfully combined e.g. 'car go', 'it hot'. Word order is not yet fixed so utterances like 'bark doggie', 'mummy where?' could be produced. Questions using question words and rising intonation are asked like 'who there?', 'daddy gone?'. Negatives are formed by using 'no' or 'not' before nouns and verbs like 'not run', 'no more'. The prepositions 'in', 'on', the word ending 'ing' as in 'boy running' are emerging. Plural 's' as in 'shoes or 'cats' is emerging. Past tense marker 'ed' as in 'baby falled' is emerging.

2-2½ years

A vocabulary of around 250 words. The beginnings of concept formation: toys, pictures and language begin to represent real objects in the child's mind. Ideas and information start to be expressed in language.

- Three element sentences like 'daddy kick ball', 'where go now', 'me want biccy', 'the red car' are now produced.
- Pronouns (I, me, you, he, she, that, this, mine, yours) begin to be used.
- Copula verb ('to be') is used as in 'I am cross', 'he is baby', 'you are big', 'cat be hurt'.
- Auxiliary verbs (have, do, may, can) with a main verb start to be used as in 'I can do', 'she is looking', 'me do like'.
- Between 2-3½ years the following word endings emerge: Past participle – I have seen / walked / talked / gone / taken / had. Third person singular 's' – he / she / it / says, walks etc. Possessive-mummy's bag, John's dog. Contracted negative – I won't / can't / don't. Contracted copula – I'm hot, he's good, daddy's here. Contracted auxiliary – I've got three, he's going home. Superlative fattest, biggest, happiest. Comparative bigger, prettier, nicer. Adverb **'ly'** – quickly, slowly, softly.

21/2 years – 3 years

Significant increase in vocabulary, now able to generalise, uses complex sentences and develops extended imaginary symbolic play sequences. Carries on simple conversations and is able to verbalise past experiences. Asks lots of questions, though many are meaningless. Words may still be simplified and telescoped. Listens to and enjoys stories, very attached to certain ones which are demanded over and over again.

- Sentences of four and more elements are used like 'Susie going to town today'. Adjectives are joined together in a sentence like, 'A big red ball'.
- Nouns and adjectives are joined by 'and' – 'boys and girls', 'wet and muddy'.
- Two auxiliary verbs may be used together – 'he will be going'.
- Uses plurals and pronouns.

3 – 31/2 years

Vocabulary continues to develop. Sentence length increases.

- Multiple sentences of more than one clause i.e. containing more than one verb are now produced. Simple statements are joined by conjunctions (and, when, because) – 'he sang and the girl danced', 'he'll come when I shout', 'he's tired because it's late'.
- Relative and nominal clauses like 'the lady who saw me', 'the box that they put it in' and clauses used as objects of the verb like 'I don't want you read that book'.
- Prepositions begin to appear.
- Comparative phrases like 'he is bigger than you' begin to be used.

31/2 – 41/2 years

Speech completely intelligible showing only a few infantile substitutions. Gives correct account of recent events and experiences, gives address and age. Asks lots of meaningful questions. Less egocentric in language, listens to and tells longer stories, confusing fact and fiction at times. Understands prepositions. Starts to know colours accurately.

- The use of auxiliary verbs is extended to include 'ought', 'might', 'should', 'must'.
- The use of passive structures begins to emerge like 'it's getting painted', 'the boy was bitten'.
- 'All', 'much', 'both', 'many' appear at the beginning of a noun phrase – 'all the people', 'both my sisters'.
- Pronoun errors like 'her doing it' still occur.

41/2 + years

- The different types of comparative such as 'prettier' versus 'more beautiful' are learned.
- Sentence connecting devices and comment clauses like 'actually', 'you know', and fillers like 'sort of' begin to be used.
- The child may not fully understand: passive sentences, subordinating conjunctions (although, unless, since) verbs like 'promise', 'ask', 'tell', adjectives like 'eager to', 'easy to', 'hard to' and 'anxious to'.

5 years

A vocabulary of around 1,500-2,000 words. Prepositions used appropriately and to give directions. 'Why' questions asked and responses listened to. Speech generally more fluent and accurate; however, confusion with fricatives (s, f, th) often still remains. Refers to concrete nouns by use and asks the meaning of abstract words. Language is much more purposeful. Loves stories and will act them out, live them.

6 years

A vocabulary of around 3,000 words, with good articulation. Use of verb tenses, past and future, emerging with a degree of accuracy (future concept is harder than that of the past). Beginning to be able to relate ideas and understand cause and effect. Interested in written language and able to relate own experiences to those in books.

Language development continues after the age of six in a number of important areas. Vocabulary and word-meaning expansion are the most obvious aspects of later language development but other high-level language skills are important:

- comprehending beyond the actual words in a text (inference).
- understanding a range of colloquial terms.
- understanding double and implied meanings.
- understanding puns, plays on words and jokes.
- more complex spelling and grammar skills.

Failure to expand language competence beyond the basic level reached at six can frequently pass unnoticed. There are important consequences however, for intellectual development and for learning and performance in school.

The development of pragmatic skills – the use of language for social interaction

First few months of life – eye contact established between mother and child.

3 months – child's gaze follows adult's, leading to joint attention of other objects. Parents and carers respond to the child's noises as if they are intentional communication which establishes an early basis for dialogue and later conversation.

3-6 months – turn-taking games like 'peekaboo' develop – these are important for facilitating parent-child interaction, and adults start including nearby objects and actions in these to-and-fro language games. This relies heavily on shared attention and eye contact to associate words and things.

12+ months – as the child's language emerges, more vocalisation than gesture is used. Conversation starts and from one-year onwards children begin to consciously play with language, using silly voices for animals etc.

2-3 years – children develop linguistic strategies in order to gain attention – they use focusing remarks to prepare someone else for action, e.g. Child; 'You see that train.' adult: 'Yes.' child:'Well, I want it.'

They also try out language games on parents. They make, and can respond to, simple requests and can make statements or comments. They become increasingly aware of the social functions of communication and begin to learn to negotiate. At two, this may simply mean pushing another child out of the way and grabbing the bike!

By **3 years** – children have generally acquired the ability to make and respond to clarification requests, and stylistic variations of language are heard in role-play (e.g. they use features of 'Daddy's' speech when pretending to be Daddy).

By **4 years** – children are beginning to 'read between the lines', i.e. to perceive the intention behind the speech. For example, they can understand reasoned responses, e.g. Child: 'Can I go out now?' Adult: 'It's raining. Why not play with the train?'

There is an increased capacity to joke and to lie. Children at this age can learn in a group of other children and can negotiate with others, using language to sort out problems and to build on prior learning.

By **4 to 6 years** – children are able to hold quite complicated conversations. The following skills are appearing and continue to develop as the child grows up.

● They can see when a conversation is breaking down and request clarification or try to repair the conversation; 'Did you mean that one?' or 'What do you mean?'

- They can join and finish a conversation appropriately, using non-verbal and verbal strategies: making or breaking eye contact, saying 'Can I just say this?' or 'Thanks, bye'.
- They can assess and use knowledge of different social contexts and personal characteristics and use appropriate body language, gesture, tone of voice and expression. They can adjust to others' moods and levels of interest.
- They can refer back to the past and forward to the future and use world knowledge, showing understanding of colloquialisms, jokes, puns, etc.

Stages in speech sound development

( ) = sound just beginning to appear, but inconsistent.

Stage	Sounds involving lips	Sounds involving tongue	Sounds at back of mouth
1 1½-2 years	m p b w	n t d	
2 2-2½ years	m p b w	n t d	(ing) (k g) h
3 2½-3½ years	m p b f w	n t d s (l) y	ing k g h
4 3½-4 years	m p b f v w	n t d ch j sh s z l (r) y	ing k g h
5 4½ + years	m p b f v w	n t d ch j th sh s z l r y	ing k g h

Sound production development

	50% of children by	90% of children by
p m h n w	1y 6m	3y
b	1y 6m	4y
k g d	2y	4y
t ng	2y	6y
f y	2y 6m	4y
r l	3y	6y
s	3y	6y
sch h	3y 6m	7y
z	4y	7y
j	4y	7y
v	4y	8y
th	4y 6m	7y
th (the)	5y	8y
s (measure)	6y	8y 6m

First Words

These are key words chosen from across the curriculum.
At first children may give one word answers before moving to simple sentences. The next stage sees the introduction of longer structures and a wider vocabulary.

Prompts:Who/what is this? Who/what is that? Who's this? Who's that?

Replies: This is That is That's It's

Animals

Pets – fish bird rabbit mouse
Garden – butterfly worm snail ladybird spider
Farm – horse cow chicken pig sheep duck goat
Zoo – monkey bear polar bear elephant lion tiger zebra snake giraffe seal

Body parts

head hair face eyes nose ears mouth lips teeth tongue neck cheeks shoulders arm hand fingers thumbs leg elbow feet toes knee tummy/stomach chest back wrist ankle

Clothes

pants vest shirt tie socks tee-shirt tights trousers shorts skirt dress cardigan jumper shoes pumps trainers coat hat scarf gloves

Colours

red orange yellow green blue black white purple pink grey brown silver gold

Drink

milk juice lemonade pop tea coffee

Feelings

happy sad cross/angry good naughty bad hungry thirsty tired
(Who is…? Dad is Dad is happy Dad's happy)

Food

Fruit – apple banana orange pear strawberry lemon plum grape tomato
Vegetable – potato cabbage onion carrot beans peas
Meat – chicken sausage burger
Other – cheese bread butter biscuit

Numbers

1 2 3 4 5 6 7 8 9 10
a little bit, a lot, more, all of it, some, another, any, any more, many, some more, anymore, no more, less/fewer, as much as, as many as, equals, altogether

(How many? How much? How many more/less?)

first, second, third, fourth, fifth, sixth, seventh, eighth, ninth, tenth
first, next, last, at the front, at the back
(Where is the../ Which one is...?)

People/Family

Mum/mummy Dad/daddy boy girl baby man woman people
family brother sister friend nana/nain/gran grandad/taid

Other nouns

cat dog house car tree bed book ball doll teddy egg flower cake
box apple cup sweet balloon

Positions

in on under behind in front open/shut/closed up/down top/
bottom over off out next to/by between against far/near corner/
middle/edge

(Where is the cat? On the chair. It's on the chair.)

Same / Different

noisy, loud/quiet high/low hard/soft wet/dry hot/cold rough/
smooth big/little long/short tall/short fat/thin heavy/light full/
empty fast/slow early/late today/yesterday/tomorrow
(Which is...? Which one is...?This one That one)

Shapes

circle square rectangle triangle dot star straight/curved line

Vehicles

Road – car bus van lorry bike
Rail – train
Air – plane helicopter rocket
Water – boat ship submarine

Verbs

Running, walking, jumping, skipping, crying, laughing, sleeping,
awaking, drinking, eating, working, playing, standing, sitting, falling,
lying down, reading, writing, dancing, swimming, painting, drawing,
getting, picking, holding, making, cutting, sticking/gluing,
fastening/fixing together, looking, washing, drying, listening,
thinking,
(What is the boy doing? Who is running?
The boy's running. The boy is running.
What are you doing? What is he/she doing, etc.)

Next Stage

This covers the first words vocabulary but with longer, more complex or different structures. Then, the additional vocabulary is introduced. It should be noted that the pace of introduction is governed by the pupil/pupils' readiness and progress. There may be many weeks' work in one section.

Answering questions with yes/no

E.g. Is mum walking? Is the cat fat? Is it hot? Is this rough? Is he wet?

Extending utterances using conjunctions and/or

E.g. The boy is running and jumping. Who is running and jumping? Is the boy walking or running? The house is big and red. What is big and red? Is it small? He is wearing shorts and a tee-shirt. Who is wearing shorts and a tee-shirt? What is he wearing?

Using simple plurals

E.g. The cats are running. What are they doing? Are they sleeping? Mum and dad are working. What are they doing?

Using verb patterns

With past tense mostly regular 'ed' verbs but others as they arise naturally in conversation/activities.
E.g. What are you going to do? I am /I'm going to paint.
What are you doing? I am/I'm painting.
What did you do? I painted a picture.
Who did you see? I saw grandma.

Using was/were

E.g. What was he doing? He was writing. She was good. They were busy.

Using negatives

E.g. can/can't, do/don't, is/isn't, has/hasn't, have/haven't
He isn't coming. She is. She can't hop. No I can't. Do you want some? No I don't. I don't like milk. I do like cheese.

Using possessives

E.g. Whose coat is this? Emma's coat. Steven's. It's Emma's. It's his. It's hers. Itself. Themselves.

Irregular plurals

E.g. scarves chidren men/women mice
Extending with conjunctions so/because

Irregular past tense

E.g. came, gave, put, went, sat, took, ran, had, made, found, broke, fell, built

Verb negatives

E.g. am not/I'm not, aren't/ are not, hasn't, haven't, didn't, doesn't, wasn't, won't, weren't

Irregular past tense

E.g. ate, blew, bought, brought, chose, drank, drew, dug, read, rode, slept, spent, stood, swung

Future verbs with 'will'

We will go outside after lunch. They will come to tea on Sunday.

Irregular unchanging plurals

E.g. sheep, deer, fish

Irregular past participles with 'has'

E.g. blown, broken, chosen, come, drawn, driven, drunk, eaten, fallen, flown, given, gone, run, taken, thrown

Using would/should/could/might

Additional vocabulary

Animals

Parts – tail, whiskers, tusk, paws, claws, beak, wings, horn
Babies – foal, piglet, calf, chick, duckling, lamb, kitten, puppy
Homes – stable, pigsty, field, barn, pond, hutch, tank, nest, hive, hole, kennel

Body parts

Nostrils, eyelashes, eyebrows, skin, knuckles

Clothes

Fastenings – zip, buckle, hooks, buttons, Velcro, laces, belt, PE kit, pumps

Colour

dark/light/pale darker/lighter shades

Food

Raspberry, blackberry, satsuma, pineapple, rice, spaghetti, jelly, ice-cream, hot/cold food/drinks, fizzy/still

People

Twins, cousins, aunts, uncles, nephew, niece, teacher, headteacher/ head, secretary, cook, cleaner, caretaker, dinner lady, taxi driver policeman, doctor, dentist

Shapes

Oval, diamond, hexagon, pentagon, sphere, cube, pyramid, cone

Vehicles

Scooter, raft, tricycle, jet, yacht, hovercraft
Parts – lights, wings, wheel, steering-wheel, propeller

Adjectives

sharp/blunt, silky, furry, squashy, stretchy, quick/slow, jerky/smooth, thin/thick, wide/narrow, deep/shallow, dirty/clean, pretty/lovely/ugly, nice/awful, shiny/dull, plastic/metal/wood/glass/fabric, natural/manmade, see-through [transparent]/opaque, magnetic/not magnetic, electrical, waterproof, strong, push/pull, living/dead, moving, bending, twisting, stretching, melting/freezing, right/wrong, broken/mended, tidy/untidy, loose/tight, sweet/sour, strong/weak, poor/rich, real/not real/imaginary, kind/unkind, tired/energetic, clever/stupid, silly/sensible, careful/dangerous, pleased, surprised, frightened, worried, better/worse ill/poorly/sick/well

Use of comparatives 'er'/ 'est'
Where?

Along, forwards/backwards, sideways, through, across, above/below, back/front, upstairs/downstairs, at, to, from, about, beside, together, around, apart, towards/away from, inside/outside, into/out of, opposite/facing, anywhere/everywhere/nowhere/somewhere, here, there

When?

Before/after, afterwards, now, later, then, evening/night/day, old/new, old/young, once, suddenly, again, sometime, long ago, while, already, until, always, yet, soon, since, almost, nearly, usually, often, o'clock/half past, etc., dinner/home/play time

How many?

most/least, fewest, part, several, whole, together, the rest, plenty, enough, only, each, either, anything/everything/nothing/something, anybody/nobody/everybody/somebody, a pair, both

Verbs

Kneeling, clapping, hopping, climbing, singing, shouting, whispering, pretending, trying to, pulling/pushing, waiting, coming, going, hurrying, staying, turning, starting/stopping, leaving, teaching, helping, seeing, digging, flying, riding, diving, growing, fighting, winning, hiding, sewing/knitting,
Put, stick, throw, say, hear, break, carry, drop, follow, mend, take, have, buy, kick, hang, kill, change, give, send, pay, show, pour, like, love, bring, catch, thank, find, lose, finish, tell, ask, watch, hit, hurt, want, keep, forget, call, smell, fill, remember, count, learn, post, knock, blow, ring, point, build, meet, mix, wear, us, know, cover, marry

Adverbs

Quickly, slowly, happily/sadly, noisily/quietly, etc.

Additional vocabulary 2

Buildings

School, castle, church, garage, hospital, library, railway, station, police station, ambulance station, fire station, museum, shop, supermarket, zoo, tent, swimming baths/pool, cinema, lighthouse, flats, office, detached/semi-detached/terraced house, bungalow

Games

Football, tennis, cricket, chase/tag, ring games, race

Garden/Park

Grass, flowers, woods/forest, bushes, weeds, leaf, gate, fence, hedge, smoke, bonfire, pond/lake, puddle, slide, swing, roundabout

Home

Rooms – kitchen, lounge/sitting room, bathroom, bedroom, toilet, hall, study
Parts – wall, door, window, floor, ceiling
Furniture – light, mat/carpet, curtain, shelf, fire, chair, table, picture, clock, cupboard, sink, cooker/oven, settee, arm/easy chair, bed, bath, toilet
Other – kettle, toaster, bowl, bucket, saucepan, cup, knife/fork/ spoon saucer, plate, teapot, jug, dish/bowl, cushion, soap, towel, toothbrush/paste, duvet/quilt, pillow, telephone

Jobs

Teacher, doctor, nurse, dentist, painter, artist, author, musician, conductor, racing/bus-driver, pilot, carpenter, mechanic, actor, shop/factory worker, zoo-keeper, therapist

Money

Names of all coins, coin, money, how much?, spend/spent, change

Seaside

Sea, sand, shell, waves, crab, bucket, spade, flag, donkey, ice-cream, funfair

Time

Days of the week, months of the year, seasons, weekend, before, after, how long, minutes/hours, o'clock/half-past/quarter to/past

Tools/equipment

Comb, tooth brush, apron, dustpan, broom, peg, needle, pin, paper-clip, drawing pin, staple, split pin, sellotape, tape, string, paper, card, pen/pencil/felt tip/crayon, box, bag/carrier bag, suitcase, torch, candle, match, spanner, screwdriver, hammer, nail, musical instruments – claves, shakers, drum, bells – computer – screen, mouse, tool bar, program, hoop, quoit, rope, bench, climbing frame, large apparatus

Weather

Frost, ice, sleet, hail, thunder, lightning, storm, rainbow, dew

Rhymes

Learning and reciting rhymes can help with:

● Developing memory skills

● Articulating particular sounds

● Using expression

● Using a loud enough voice for a group/class to hear

● Curriculum work – some of the rhymes that follow are associated with Key Stage 1 topic or curriculum work, particularly History.

Whichever particular speech sounds your pupils are working on with their speech and language therapist, be ready to praise them for a good attempt. As confidence and skill increases, expect and then praise a better attempt. For instance, if your pupil is working on /b/ then you might expect a clear / b/ at the end of /rub/ or scrub but not expect a clear /r/ or /scr/ as these are harder and will not have been practised yet. Awareness of your pupil's speech programme and of the stages of speech and language development (Appendix 1) is really helpful.

Making up alliterative phrases and sentences can be good fun, as well as providing good speaking practice. For older children, it can form part of writing and spelling tasks.

Silly Susan saw a show on Saturday.
Clever Colin caught a catfish.
Mighty Mouse made a mantrap.

Some of the rhymes we use are listed on the following pages. Some are at a simple level; others are harder with the target sound in different positions. A wider selection is given in *Phonic Rhyme Time* by Mary Nash-Wortham (LDA).

B

Bee, Bee
A bee on me!
Bzzzz

I rub and I rub
At the tub, tub, tub.
My dirty clothes
I scrub, scrub, scrub.

Bl

Black and blue
Black and blue
How are you?
I'm black and blue.

Br

New brooms!
New brooms!
Buy my brooms
to brush your rooms.
New brooms!

C

Come and play
Come and play
Can you come to my house today?

Ch

Chip chop, chip chop, chip chop Joe
Chip chop, chip chop, chip chop Joe
One big blow,
Ouch my toe!
Chip chop, chip chop, chip chop Joe

Cl

Clip clop! Clip clop!
Go and never stop
Gee up my little pony
Clip clop! Clip clop!

Cr

Crash!
Don't be cross Mum, Don't be cross.
It was an accident.
Don't be cross Mum, Don't be cross

D

Oh dear! Oh dear!
Poor Dan
Oh dear!

Have you heard about our Neddy?
Poor Ned, Poor Ned.
Have you heard about our Neddy?
Dead, dead, dead.

Dr

Careful with your drink
Don't you spill a drop
Careful with your drink
Don't let it drip, drip, drop.

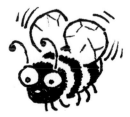

F

Jeremiah blow the fire puff, puff, puff.
Blow it gently f f f
Blow it rough fff fff fff
Jeremiah blow the fire puff, puff, puff.

Fl

There is a fly I know there is
I saw it on the floor
There is a fly I know there is
I heard it by the door.
Zzzzzzzzzzzzzzzzzzzz

Fr

5 little frogs sitting on a well
1 leaned over and down he fell
Frogs jump high
Frogs jump low
4 little frogs jump to and fro

4 little frogs sitting on a well…

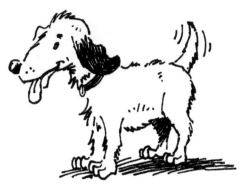

G

Go, go, go
Go fast not slow
Go, go, go

There was a little dog and he had a
little tail.
And he used to wag, wag, wag it.
But if he was sad or if he'd been bad.
Then he would drag, drag, drag it.

Gl

Glory! Glory!
I'm SO glum
I'll sit and look sad and suck my thumb.
Glory! Glory!
I'm SO glad
I'll run very fast to meet my Dad.

Gr

These are Grandma's glasses.
[Put fingers round eyes]
This is Grandma's hat.
[Put hands on head in hat shape]
Grandma claps her hands like this
And folds them in her lap.
These are Grandad's glasses.
[Put fingers round eyes]
This is Grandad's hat.
[Put hands on head in hat shape]
Grandad folds his arms like this
And has a little nap.

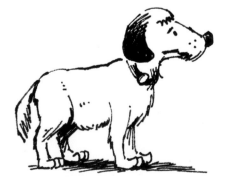

H

Here's a pieman
Hi! Hi! Hi!
Here's a penny
For a hot, hot pie.

J

Here I am little jumping Joan
Jump, jump, jump
When nobody's with me I'm all alone
Jump, jump, jump.

L

Look out! Look out!
A car is coming.
Look out! Look out!
A car is coming.
Here it comes going so fast
Just stand back and let it past
Look out! Look out!
A car is coming

M

Me, me, me
Give it to me
Me, me, me
Please

My motor is humming
I'm coming, I'm coming
Make room, make room, make room!
Not a minute to wait,
I'm late, late, late,
Make room, make room, make room!

N

No, no, no
Off you go
No, no, no

All night long when the wind is high.
Nnn Nnn Nnn Nnn
The lightships moan and moan to the sky.
The foghorns whine as the fog runs free
Warning the men in the ships at sea.
Nnn Nnn Nnn Nnn

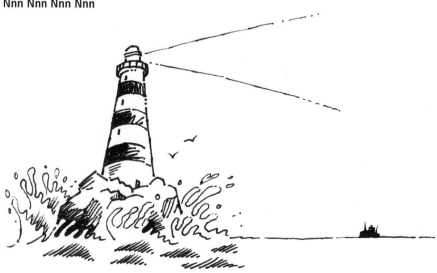

P

Pie, pie
I love pie
Pie, pie
Mmmmm!

Pease pudding hot
Pease pudding cold
Pease pudding in the pot
Nine days old.

Pr

Prick your finger princess.
Prick your finger so.
Prick your finger princess.
And off to sleep you go.

Pl

Please, please, please mum.
Plenty of peas Mum
Plenty of peas Mum
Please, please, please.

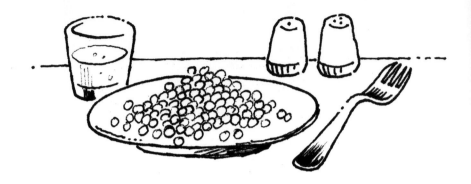

Q

Queenie, Queenie who's got the ball?
Are they short or are they tall?
Are they fat or are they thin?
Queenie, Queenie who will win?

(This is a ball game where one child
[Queenie] stands with her back to the
rest who stand in a line. Queenie
throws the ball over her shoulder and
one child catches it and hides it behind
her back. All children put hands behind
backs. Queenie turns round and they
say rhyme to her, she then guesses
who's got the ball – if right has another
go and if wrong the child with the ball
becomes Queenie.)

R

Turn rope turn.
Round and round
High in the air
And down on the ground
Turn rope turn.
Round and round.

S

A sailor went to sea, sea, sea
To see what he could see, see, see
But all that he could see, see, see
Was the bottom of the deep blue sea,
sea, sea

Sc/Sk

Here's your scarf and here's your hat
Off to school you go
Here's your bag now scat! scat! scat!
Off to school you go.

Sh

Shoe shine! Shoe shine! Shouts the
shoe shine boy.
Shoe shine! Shoe shine! Shouts the
shoe shine boy.
Shine your shoes sir!
Shine your shoes sir!
Shoe shine! Shoe shine! Shouts the
shoe shine boy.

Sl

Slugs, slugs slide so slow
Leaving silver tracks wherever they go.

Sm

If the smoke is black
Alas! Alack!
If the smoke is grey
It'll be a nice day.

Sn

Snow, snow glorious snow
On our sledges down we go
On the snow snow glorious snow.

Sp

I saw a spider spinning a web
I saw a spider crawling up the wall
I saw a spider in a sunny spot
Then he wasn't there at all.

St

The policeman's standing still in
the street
Stopping the cars just standing on
his feet
STOP! STOP! STOP!

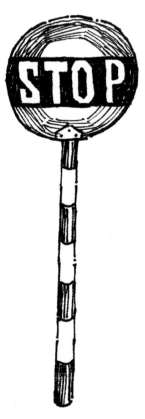

Sw

Sweep, sweep, sweep
sweep with your broom
Sweep, sweep, sweep
Sweep all of the room.

T

Our great church clock goes TICK TOCK
TICK TOCK.
Our sitting room clock goes Tick-tack
Tick-tack Tick-tack.
My little watch goes ticker-tacker,
ticker-tacker, ticker-tacker.

Th

What a thing!, I have to choose
This one or that one, that one or this
I want both but I can't have both.
This one or that one I have to choose.

Tr

Trip trap, trip trap all the way to town
Trip trap, trip trap bouncing all around.
It's not a comfy way to ride
Bouncing about from side to side
Trip trap, trip trap all the way to town.

Tw

Twenty two and twenty four
Twist the handle, open the door
Twenty six and twenty eight
Run inside I just can't wait

V

If you ever, ever, ever see a whale
You must never, never tread upon its
tail.
For if you ever, ever tread upon its tail.
You will never live to see another
whale.

W

Where does the flame on the
candle go
when you blow it out? I would
like to know.
Where does it come from and
where does it go?
That is what I would like to
know.

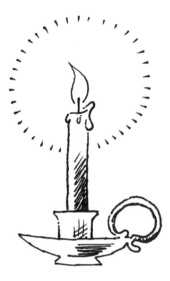

Y

Yawning [   ] is a sight
He yawns and yawns with all his might
He yawns all day and he yawns all
night
Yawning, yawning [   ]

(Put in each child's name in turn and
use he or she as appropriate.)

Z

Buzz, buzz, buzz went the busy, busy bee.
Buzz, buzz, buzz, buzz, buzz went he.

Acknowledgements:

It is impossible to give the source of all the rhymes included here. Some were jotted down while the author was searching for material for lessons. Others have been passed down orally. Every effort has been made to trace and acknowledge copyright owners. Apologies are offered to any author or copyright holder whose rights have been unintentionally infringed and due acknowledgement will be made in subsequent editions on notification being made to the publishers.

The rhymes for the following letters – B, Bl, Br, C, Cl, Cr, F, Fl, Fr, G, Gl, L, M, N, P, S, Sn, St, Sw, T, Tw, W, Y and Z – have been made up by the author or are taken or adapted from rhymes in *Speech Rhymes* edited by Clive Sansom, A & C Black (1975) ISBN 0 7136 1425 0

'Chip chop Joe' and 'These are Grandma's glasses' are taken from *This Little Puffin* compiled by Elizabeth Matterson Penguin (1969)

'Five little frogs' is taken from *One, Two, Three, Four – Number Rhymes and Finger Games* by Mary Grice. Frederick Warne (1974)

'There was a little dog' is taken from *I Never Saw A Purple Cow and other Nonsense Rhymes* by Emma Chichester Clark Walker Books (1990)

'Here I am little Jumping Joan' is taken from *Lavender's Blue – A Book of Nursery Rhymes* OUP, London (1967)

'Turn rope turn' is taken from a poem by John Agard in *Playtime Rhymes* selected by John Foster OUP (1998)

'Sand in your sandals' is taken from a poem by John Foster in *Poems for the Very Young* selected by Michael Rosen Kingfisher (1996)

The rhymes on page 15 are from *165 Chants for Children*. Edited by Mary Lou Colgin. Gryphon House Publishing (1992) and *A Child's Treasury of Milligan*. Spike Milligan, Virgin Publishing (2000)

Questions

I keep six honest serving men
They taught me all I knew;
Their names are What and Why and When
And How and Where and Who.

(From 'The Elephant's Child' in *Just So Stories* by Rudyard Kipling, Everyman Library Children's Classics. 1992)

Some children have a lot of difficulty in answering and particularly, *asking* questions. Even children without recognised speech and language difficulties can stumble when asked to devise appropriate questions. It is a skill that must be taught and practised.

At the same time, adults can find it hard to ask open-ended questions. Teachers especially, may ask a question knowing exactly the answer they want to hear from the child. When that answer is not forthcoming, they can be reluctant to accept alternatives, casting round the group until they get the 'nearest match' to the answer in their own mind, or giving up and 'putting the words into the mouths' of pupils.

It may be helpful to script questions to match the curriculum area or bank of vocabulary being worked on. Build up a bank of encouraging responses to children who have a go, but get it wrong:

'That's an interesting idea…'
'Well-tried Jason, you're on the right lines…'
'Mmm, can anyone add something else to what Poppy has said?'
'I need to think about that…'
'Thank you for that answer, Darius. Let's try and work out how you got to it. Remember, the question was…'

Teachers will be familiar with the strategy of naming the child, before asking the question, so that he is 'cued-in' and attentive. 'Kevin, can you tell us…?' It is a useful approach to share with parents.

There is an order of difficulty in questioning. **What, where** and **who** are usually easier than **when, how** and **why**. However, any kind of 'What if?' question or one that uses 'might', 'could' or 'would' is more abstract and may be as difficult as a 'Why' question.

Answering and asking questions is an important part of all curriculum work and indeed an essential life skill. The examples that follow focus on questions that may arise in design and technology work.

What?

What is it called?

What does it smell / taste / feel / sound / look like?

What size / colour is it?

What decoration does it have / what does the decoration tell you?

What lettering is there?

What is it made from / what raw materials made that?

What could be used instead of it?

What is it worth to you / to a sale room / to a man marooned on a desert island?

Where?

Where was it used / designed / made / disposed of?

Where did the museum get it from / the designer get the idea from / the materials come from?

Where would it be of most value / you keep it?

Where could you get another?

Who?

Who designed / used / made / likes / threw it away?

Who else has got one / wants one?

Who would buy it now / choose it?

Who might have bought it when it was new?

When?

When was it designed / made / used / obsolete / disposed of / altered:

When would you find it useful?

When can you try it out?

How?

How was it made / designed?

How does it work / the material affect the shape / it reflect society's attitudes or culture?

How well made / designed is it?

How well does it work?

How can it be improved / replaced?

How could it be better designed?

How would it have been made 100 years ago / you feel using it every day?

How many of them are there?

Why?

Why is it this size / shape / colour / material?

Why does it have this lettering / decoration?

Why was it made?

Why is it no longer used?

Why would anyone pay a lot of money for it?

Good listening DOs

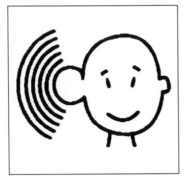

Keep listening

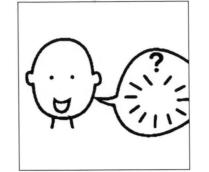

'Please say it again.'

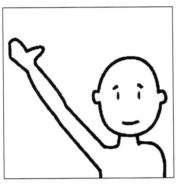

Put your hand up

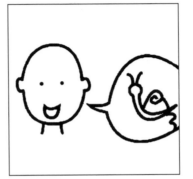

'Please say it more slowly.'

Be polite

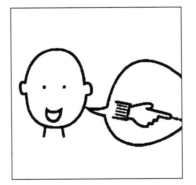

'Please show me what you mean.'

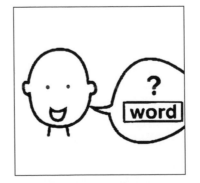

'What does that word mean?'

Good Listening pictures adapted from *Functional Language in the Classroom* by Maggie Johnson, available from the Department of Psychology and Speech Pathology, the Manchester Metropolitan University, Elizabeth Gaskell Site, Hathersage Road, Manchester M13 0JA.

Good listening DON'Ts

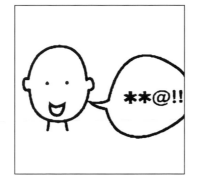

Guess without thinking first

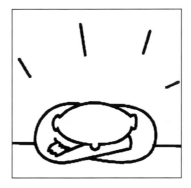

Flop

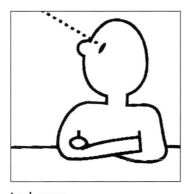

Look away

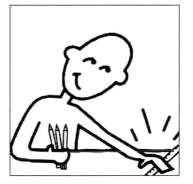

Fidget

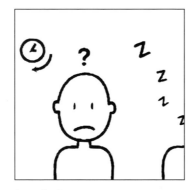

Just sit there

Change the subject

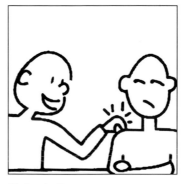

Distract others

Word Banks

The following pages may be photocopied and used to make a word-bank book. The word wall is produced as a blank copy on page 104 for you to write in fewer and/or different words as appropriate.

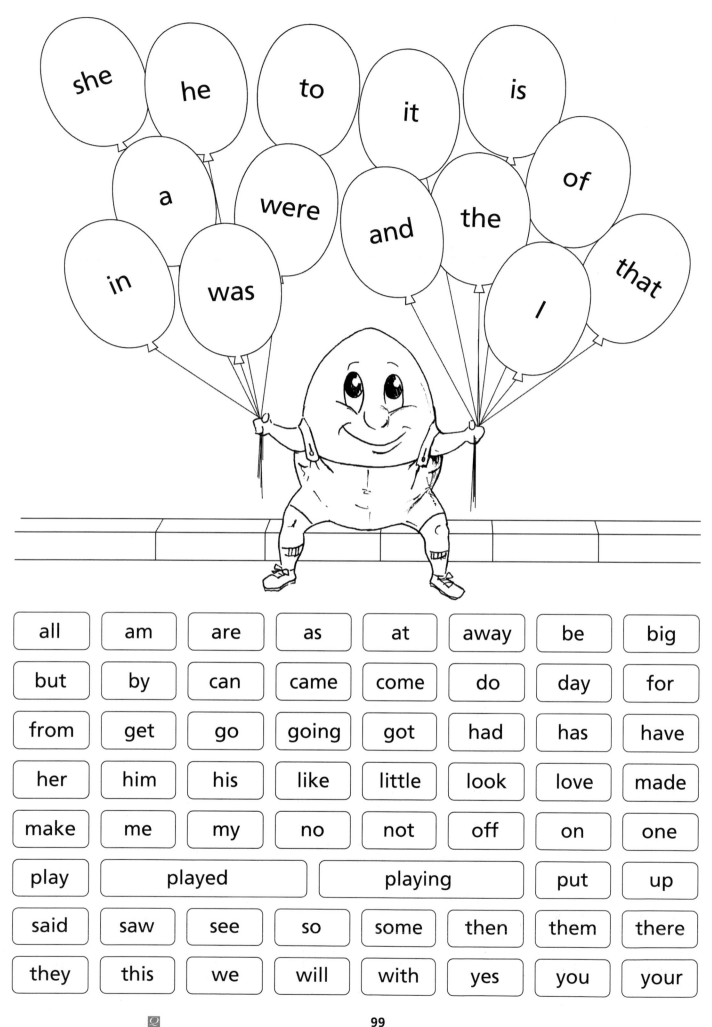

she he to it is

a were and the of

in was I that

all	am	are	as	at	away	be	big
but	by	can	came	come	do	day	for
from	get	go	going	got	had	has	have
her	him	his	like	little	look	love	made
make	me	my	no	not	off	on	one
play	played		playing		put	up
said	saw	see	so	some	then	them	there
they	this	we	will	with	yes	you	your

giant	monster	dragon	witch	old woman
old man	dinosaur	little boy	little girl	cat
dog	ghost	robot	queen	king
princess	prince	house	cottage	castle

palace	cave	volcano	one	red
			two	orange
			three	yellow
			four	green
			five	blue
hole	tent	tree house	six	pink
			seven	purple
			eight	black
			nine	white
			ten	brown

big little	fat thin	rich poor	happy sad cross	lonely friend	beautiful handsome ugly	lots	grey
						hundred	silver
Once One day Once upon a time		there		was lived		more	gold
						not many	blond

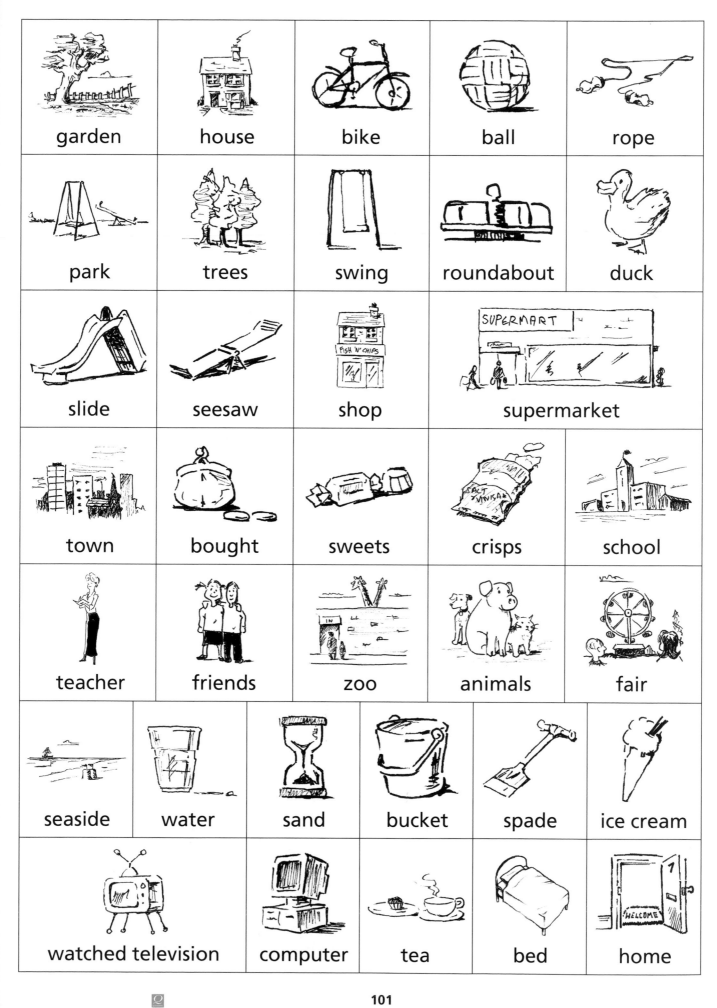

garden	house	bike	ball	rope
park	trees	swing	roundabout	duck
slide	seesaw	shop	supermarket	
town	bought	sweets	crisps	school
teacher	friends	zoo	animals	fair
seaside	water	sand	bucket	spade	ice cream
watched television	computer	tea	bed	home

	Aa	
	Bb	
	Cc	
	Ch ch	
	Dd	
	Ee	
	Ff	
	Gg	
	Hh	
	Ii	
	Jj	
	Kk	
	Ll	
	Mm	
	Nn	

	Oo	
	Pp	
	Qq	
	Rr	
	Ss	
	Sh sh	
	Tt	
3	Th th	
	Uu	
	Vv	
	Ww	
	Xx	
	Yy	
	Zz	

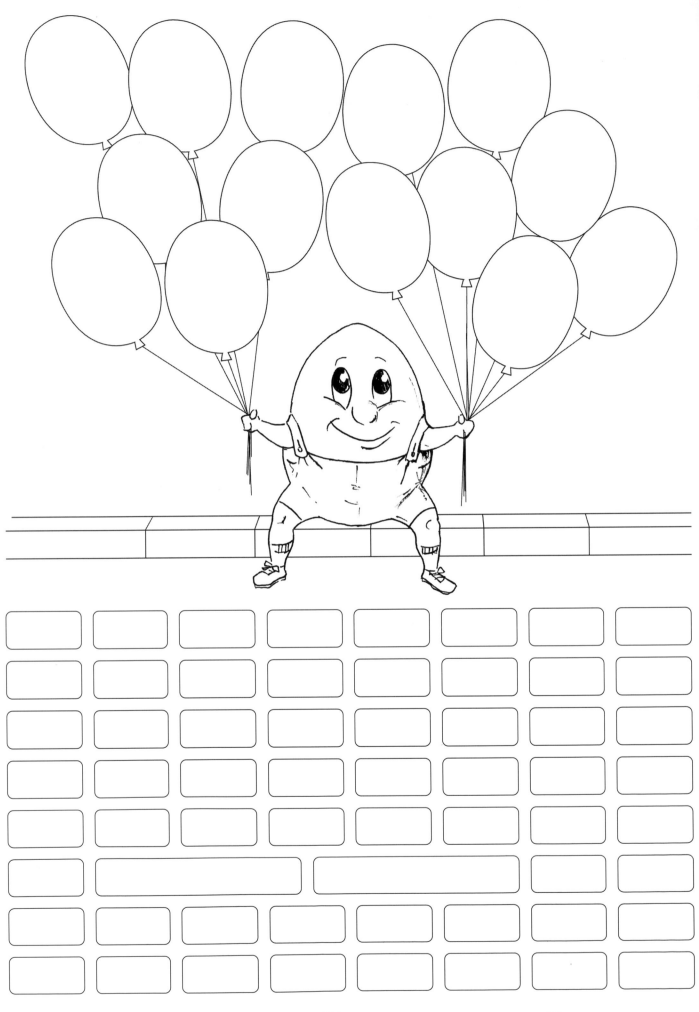

Calendars

Construct a simple calendar that a child could use at home, use blutack to move the yesterday/today/tomorrow along. Put in personal key events – school days and home days, Rainbows, swimming etc.

Some children may need the calendar broken down into the 'number of sleeps' rather than, or as well as, the days, so draw in a sun and a bed on each day.

Monday	Tuesday	Wednesday	Thursday	Friday	Saturday	Sunday
Yesterday	Today	Tomorrow				

As children become confident, a more detailed version can be used. Draw in the events, especially ones for which equipment from home has to be taken into school – recorders, PE, swimming etc.

	Monday	Tuesday	Wednesday	Thursday	Friday	Saturday	Sunday
Morning

breakfast | | | | | | | |
| Afternoon

lunch | | | | | | | |
| Evening

tea | | | | | | | |

It may be useful to have a whole-year calendar that is all on view all the time. Put in special events like birthdays and Christmas etc.

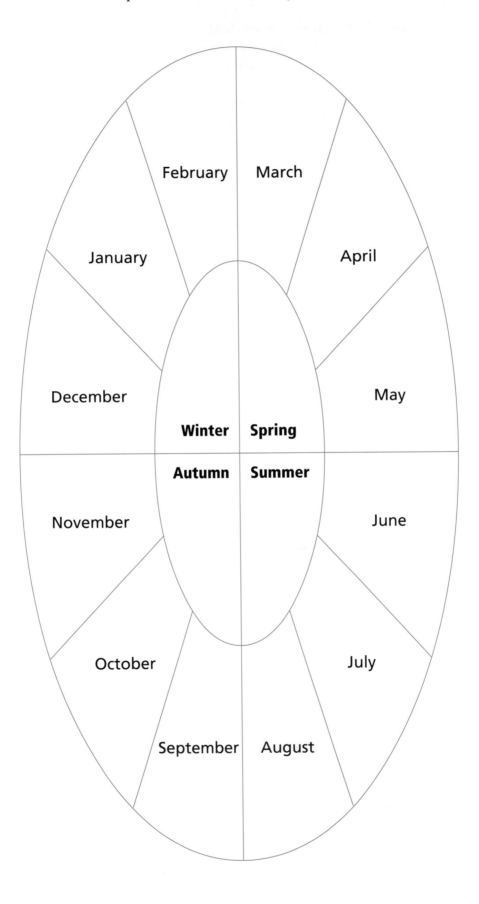

How can you help your child?

There is a great deal that parents, carers and other family members can do to help a child with speech and language difficulties. You will help your child by just 'being there' for him; listening to him, talking to him, showing him that you are interested in what he says and does and proud of his achievements, no matter how small they are.

The single most important requirement in terms of development, is your child's self-confidence. Help him to believe in himself and have the confidence to try.

Avoid talking to other adults about your child's difficulties in front of him – it will only reinforce his feeling that he is a 'problem'. Help his brothers and sisters, grandma and grandad to understand how to help as well. There are some ideas below – you will think of many more yourself, because you know your child better than anyone else.

The home is an ideal place to provide a wide range of experiences in a secure and loving setting:

At mealtimes ask your child to put the peelings in the bin, or to lay the table. You could talk about:

- **Utensils** – cutlery, pots, pans, etc., what they are called, what they are made of, what they are used for.
- **Food** – where it was grown, how it got to the shop, what sort of shop, how it was prepared, how it was cooked, its colour, its shape, its texture, its taste.
- **Positions** – who is sitting next to whom, opposite whom, at the top of the table, on the left or the right.
- **Time** – what time it is when you eat, morning, afternoon, evening, late, early, what you did first, second, etc., what you did before the meal and what you will do after the meal, what you always do at mealtimes and what you never do.

It should be an enjoyable time so make a game out of it. Perhaps take it in turns to say one thing about an object or play 'I spy something made of metal', or sing the names of the food to a tune you both know. Choose one thing at a time rather than try to do everything at once.

Rhymes, songs and stories are beneficial for many reasons: rhythm, listening, remembering, labelling, answering questions, vocabulary, eye contact, turn-taking and having fun. You can enjoy these in the bath, at bedtime, waiting for the bus or driving along in the car.

Homemade scrap books and photograph albums with photographs of the child himself and other family members are great for learning vocabulary and extending language. He can add drawings, labels and tickets from trips out, programmes from the pantomime etc.

General guidance

Reward your child for his efforts. Whatever the quality of your child's speech and language, reward a good try, pay attention, smile, touch, praise and repeat back what has been said. Of course if you know your child can do a little better with some positive encouragement then give some but do make allowances for tiredness, lack of confidence and bad days. If your child has difficulty talking, give him time and encouragement.

Speak clearly. It is important that your child hears you using good clear language. Your own speech can be simplified and used alongside gesture to gear down to the child's level of understanding. When the child makes a mistake, try one of these approaches rather than simply correcting him.

Restating:	child — 'dog'
	adult —'yes, look the **horse** is running,'
	Gently point out the correct word then find opportunities to use it a lot.
Expanding:	child —'car, car'
	adult —'yes, it's a police car and it's going fast'
Prompting:	adult —'it's not a dog it's a ...'
	child —'horse'
	adult —'well remembered, the horse is ... '
Recasting:	child —'horse likes grass'
	adult —'yes, the horse is eating grass. <pause> Grass is good food for horses.'

In this way you have repeated back what the child has said, making him feel good but you've changed it just enough to reinforce a word you're practising (horse) and you've introduced some new language (food).

If your child is passive and rarely starts talking or rarely responds, try:

● Responding enthusiastically to any reaction from him whether it's a sound or a gesture or just a glance at you.
● Repeating the sound or gesture and telling him it is good that he is joining in.
● Using favourite routines and nursery rhymes until he responds in some way.

The less a child talks the more opportunities and encouragement are needed.

If your child stutters there are some ways you can help. Don't focus on the stuttering or label your child as a stutterer. Don't ask him to slow down or try to think about what he is saying. Try not to finish sentences for him. Do give him the same chances to talk as everyone else in the family and give him time. Make sure he has his turn in family talk and doesn't have to fight to be heard. Listen to what he says and answer or comment on that, not to how he says it. Notice which situations seem to worry your child and be ready to help him.

This could be when visitors come or when he is questioned directly, for instance.

If your child has difficulty understanding you can help by making sure he is looking at you and you have his full attention. Use words your child knows. Use short, simple sentences. Try and talk about what is happening or has only just happened. Try to make talking good fun and so increase your child's confidence.

Try to choose good times to practise when neither you nor your child is too tired. Remember, if given a few pointers, other family members will probably be keen to help. Grandparents or older brothers and sisters can provide different ways of practising whilst having fun. 'Little and often' is a good rule of thumb.

Avoid outbursts of frustration by finding ways for your child to release pent-up energy in activity like football, swimming, catch, walking, bike riding, gardening, dusting or polishing. Many parents find the time just after their child gets home from school is difficult. Talk with the teacher and plan some activities with your child, to establish a routine for arriving home.

Good manners: parents and other family members can also help specifically with the demonstration of acceptable social codes and behaviour such as taking turns and saying 'please' and 'thank you'.

You can help your child develop his memory by sending him to fetch things and by giving him messages to take to other family members in and around the house. If he needs a lot of help with this at first, give very short messages and if necessary draw a little picture for him to carry in case he forgets, or write the words down if he can read them. You can very gradually lengthen the messages or the distance or time over which he will try to remember.

Friends are important. Help your child to make and develop friendships. School can be a lonely place without friends and the world outside school even lonelier. It may mean extra effort in overseeing friendships by inviting friends round, arranging outings to the park, etc. and supervising these more closely than for other children. Rainbows, Beavers, Brownies, Cubs, dance classes, gym classes and swimming classes have all proved helpful and enjoyable for some children. It is sometimes advisable to have a private word with the group organiser first and explain the kinds of difficulties your child might have. They are usually most understanding.

Many children with speech and language difficulties find friendships difficult and are vulnerable because of this. They can become targets for bullying. One way to deal with this is to build up a good group of friends who will support and look after each other.

What's wrong with him?

It can be difficult to know what to say when friends and neighbours ask what's wrong with your child. Do think it through before someone asks, though, and choose a way of explaining that is comfortable for you. Here are some suggestions that have worked for other parents:

- My son is bright and able but he has a particular difficulty with language.
- She needs help to learn to speak clearly.
- He needs help to understand language.
- If you're not understanding her don't worry, I don't sometimes. Try asking her to show you or just leave it and perhaps say, "I know you are working hard to talk more clearly and I will be able to understand you better soon if you keep on working hard."
- If you think he is not understanding don't worry, try saying it again more simply by 'chunking' what you're saying into shorter sentences with pauses in between.
- Please carry on talking with her because she enjoys talking with you and it helps her.

Some suggestions for games

- **Kim's game**:- Prepare a tray of 5 or 6 small items. Give the child a chance to look at them then cover the tray and remove one item. Ask, "What is missing?" you can gradually increase the number of items that are removed and that have to be remembered. Or use a magazine picture with a number of items, look at it then cover it and try to remember as many items as you can.

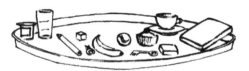

- Arrange 2 or 3 items in order. Have the child close his eyes while you mix them up. Can he put them back in order? You can do the same with a few coloured crayons or blocks.
- Write 3 numbers or letters then cover them up. Can he write them on his paper?
- Cut up the simple comic strip stories from a child's comic and have him put them in order and tell the story.
- Complete jigsaws making sure you guide your child to look for pieces that fit together because of their shape, colour or what item or part item is on them. If your child finds jigsaws difficult, give him an almost-completed puzzle, with two or three pieces missing and let him try to complete it. Gradually increase the number of missing pieces.
- Help to develop memory by playing games where your child has to listen and then do several actions. Example: Hop to the door, touch the floor, turn round twice and sit down.
- Give your child 3 or 4 items in a pile then call out an order. When you've finished speaking he has to put the items in that order. Let

him have a turn at telling you as well. You can do this with numbers, letters and words.

- I went to the shop and I bought... Usually in this game players choose an item in turn, following the letters of the alphabet (apple, banana, carrot, date, egg...) You could adapt it by giving different categories e.g. food, shapes, animals, tools... and play as above or have a maximum number of items to be remembered.
  First player: I went to the shops and I bought a sandwich.
  Second player: I went to the shops and I bought a sandwich and a bag of crisps.
  Third player: I went to the shops and I bought a sandwich, a bag of crisps and some biscuits etc...
- Rhymes: use currently popular songs or nursery rhymes. Sing or say them, leaving a pause for your child to give the rhyming word (Baa, baa, black sheep have you any wool? Yes sir, yes sir, three bags _____.) (Uh-oh, I'm in trouble, someone's come along and they burst my _____), etc. Or make up your own, like this – I'm thinking of something that rhymes with bun. It shines in the sky. It is the _____.
- I-Spy: play the original by all means (I spy something beginning with ...) but also it can be adapted for almost any language work. "I spy something rough/smooth, big/small, a vehicle, something that's red ..."
- Read a short story and after your child has listened to it, he can tell it to you or draw pictures in order. This can also be done with well-known or favourite stories.

Old favourites – Don't forget all the usual activities and games that are valuable and fun.

- Read to your child. Sit side by side sometimes so that your child can see the text and see your finger moving along under the print. Ask what might happen next or, with a longer story, recap the story so far each time you read a chapter.
- Watch television together. There are some really interesting programmes these days and some parents have found a selection of videos on colour, animals, vehicles, etc. really helpful. Then you will have a shared context to talk about.
- Hunt the Thimble, Snakes and Ladders and Ludo are all good for practising position words and the Hokey Cokey is great for left and right. Snap and Dominoes help develop careful looking.
- Puzzles books and comics may have dot to dot, mazes and colouring; fun ways to practise pencil control. Comics and puzzle books also have pictures to talk about and spot the difference games that are excellent for language work and fun to do.
- Some children need to practise balancing, running, jumping and other movement skills. Bike riding and ball games are outdoor fun and skills that some of our children need to practise a lot. Swimming is an excellent and fun activity. Some children have been greatly helped by going to a gym club.

Older children

As children grow up and strive to become more independent, it is important to help them help themselves. Some simple equipment can be a big help:

- A smart filofax in which to jot things down that may otherwise be forgotten, such as party invitations, trips, etc. It can also contain vital information like personal addresses, phone numbers, dates of birth and emergency plans for who to phone and where to go when things go wrong.
- A very small cassette recorder if jotting things down is difficult because of writing and handwriting problems.
- If appropriate AFASIC produce a smart, unobtrusive plastic card that briefly but clearly explains the holder's difficulties with language.
- A clear pencil case so the contents are visible. Two sets of pens, ruler etc. one for homework, one for school.
- A talking watch, available from The RNIB, PO Box 173, Peterborough, PE2 6WS.

Discuss with your child how in some situations some people will not understand them and maybe your child will not understand what they mean either. Discuss possible strategies;

- "I'm not very good with words."
  "I don't understand."
  "Could you write it down please?"
  "Can you tell me another way please?"
  "I'll just leave it for now thank you."
- Phone home for help. Teach them to always check that they have coins for the phone and/or a phone card. As a back-up, teach them how to make a reverse charge call.
- Sometimes in peer group situations, it may be best to walk away.

When giving instructions say them more than once, then have your child repeat them back to you. If there is quite a lot of information to remember try to make it as simple as possible.

- Encourage your child to repeat the instruction silently to himself while on the way to do it.
- Try using visual imagery (pictures in the mind) to help the memory. If your child is sent to buy milk, bread and a newspaper, make it clear there are three things to remember, then make a funny picture like reading the paper with a glass of milk in one hand and a sandwich in the other.
- Try using pictures, maps and diagrams as well.
- Sticky note pads are excellent for this as they can be stuck up for a time, then removed easily when not needed.
- Most importantly, have the children make up or choose their own ways of remembering and have them write their own reminder notes and lists. In this way they will become more self-reliant.

School survival

Children need to consider, what difficulties they are having and how they can use their strengths to help themselves in different contexts: general organisation, working in class, breaktimes, homework and exams.

- Instead of parents remembering and packing games kit, swimming kit, etc. children should learn to do so themselves. Have a weekly timetable in a conspicuous place and check it at a regular time every day. (See page 36.)
- It is useful to carry a basic tool kit that includes pens, calculator, inhaler, etc. and it should be the child's responsibility to organise replacements.
- In class, children need to think about sitting in a good place in the room to help them with their work. This might mean away from the distractions of the window or near to the middle where they can hear and see well. They need to make sure there is enough space on the table or desk to get out what is needed. Then settle down to listen and remember to look at the teacher when she is speaking.
- Discuss a range of strategies for breaks and lunchtimes. What are the rules and procedures for these times? Discuss strategies for joining a group, leaving a group and possible responses to current peer group jargon. What is the dinner menu? Discuss possible choices.
- Bullying can sometimes occur for a variety of reasons. Some children are not good at fast peer group talk, which can change rapidly as new words, and phrases come into fashion. They may have difficulty following the rules of current games and may not understand jokes. This makes them vulnerable. One of the best ways round this is to have a good friend or friends. Although you cannot force particular children to be your child's friend, you can help by being involved in their social life. You can encourage and support through being a willing taxi, giving invitations home to tea, and invitations to come on trips and by being aware which after-school clubs or groups it might be helpful for your child to join.
- Homework is something else that needs organising. Your child will benefit from you taking an interest in his homework and sometimes, helping him with it. Even if you don't know a lot about science or history, just helping him to understand the task and plan out his work, will be of benefit. Most schools have a homework jotter in which the homework task is listed, with the handing-in date. It is essential for children to use this conscientiously.
- It is helpful to have homework partners or at least have the phone numbers of one or two reliable friends who are doing the same homework.
- It may be possible to put some homework onto tape rather than writing all assignments or for your child to dictate for you to write. Such possibilities need to be discussed with the school.
- Children should not be spending long hours on homework every night and if this becomes the case, then the situation needs to be discussed with the school.

Make sure you have the name and number of a member of staff who is your contact person at the school. Then, if you have any queries or something goes wrong you have an immediate contact.

Parental faith and support are probably the most important things that any parent can give their child. So, apart from the practical ideas given above, try and keep a positive attitude. That and a sense of humour will see you through.

What the words really mean

Speaking and speech

Articulation	Movement of the tongue, jaws, soft palate and lips to make sounds
Cluttering	Speech not fluent, often too fast, words pushed together
Consonants ('C')	Sounds made by some kind of tongue or lip closure
Consonant clusters, mixes or blends	More than one consonant occurring next to each other (plant, small)
s blends **l blends** **r blends** **digraphs**	sc, sk, sl, sm, sn, sp, st, sw bl, cl, fl, gl, pl, sl br, cr, dr, fr, gr, pr, tr sh, ch, th, wh, qu
C.V.C.	Consonant - Vowel - Consonant (cat, pin, leg, etc.)
Cued articulation	A signing system, designed by a speech and language therapist, to support the production of speech sounds
Dysarthria, dysarthric	Muscle weakness in the speech muscles, causing speech patterns to be abnormal because the muscles cannot be moved correctly for speech
Dysfluent	Jerky, uneven speech
Dysphonia, dysphonic	Impaired voice, it may be gruff, husky or squeaky
Dyspraxia, dyspraxic, articulatory dyspraxia	The speech muscles can move correctly but messages to move them are not getting through from the brain, causing abnormal speech
Intelligible speech	Speech that is clear, easy to understand
Unintelligible speech	Speech that is not clear, difficult to understand
Phonology/phonological	The sounds that make up a word
Phonological awareness	Awareness/recognition of letter sounds in different positions in words
Phonological/ articulatory disorder	Difficulty making speech sounds – some may be incorrect and some may be missing
Phonological programming difficulty	Difficulty remembering and recalling letter sounds in the right order
Phoneme	A single sound (cat)
Phonemic substitution	One sound is replaced by another (tat for cat)
Phonetics	Writing how a word is pronounced
Prosody, inflection, expression	The music of speech, how it sounds. The way speech goes up and down, louder and quieter, faster and slower and is stressed and unstressed
Stuttering/stammering	Speech not fluent, jerky. Speaker may get stuck on certain sounds, especially the first sound in a word and repeat these over and over or be unable to say them
Vowels ('V')	Sounds made by lip movement and an open mouth

Language

Alternative/augmentative communication	Something used in place of or to support speech (typewriter, computer, symbol system (like Rebus) or signing system (like Paget Gorman or cued articulation). Any form of Augmentative communication is not a language in its own right
Asperger's Syndrome	Autistic children who have more language, mix better and learn more. They may be clumsy, eccentric, etc. But seem to do better than other autistic children
Autism	Children with autism will have constant difficulties mixing, talking and playing with others. Play can be very repetitive and behaviour can be eccentric and obsessive
Autistic spectrum continuum Pervasive developmental disorders	All kinds of autism including Asperger's and semantic pragmatic difficulties
Concepts	Meanings behind the word labels (hot/cold, rough/smooth, more/one more/a lot more/many, etc.)
Dyslexia/specific learning difficulties	Children who, though intelligent, have difficulty with reading and writing
Elective/selective mutism	Children who choose not to speak in some situations or with some people
Expressive language	The production of words and sentences, the actual talking
Expressive language delay Developmental language delay Specific language delay	When a child is not talking as much, in number of words or sentences and in complexity of sentences, as other children of the same age
Expressive language disorder Developmental language disorder Specific language difficulty Specific language impairment Developmental aphasia Developmental dysphasia	Unclear, limited language. A child is unable to explain what he or she means in a way that others can understand. When language develops it does not follow a normal pattern
High level language disorder	Understanding simple, straightforward language but not more complex language like double meanings, hidden meanings, sayings, colloquialisms, humour or structures like "I ought to", "except". Interpreting language literally
Language development	The expected number of words, sentences, length of sentence and complexity of sentence for each age group
PGSS or Paget Gorman Signing System	A signing system (not a language) that can be used to support language development
Pragmatics	Knowing what to say, when to say it and how to say it to other people
Receptive language/ comprehension	Understanding what is said
Receptive language disorder/ difficulty	Not understanding what is said

SALT/SLT	Speech And Language Therapist
Semantics	The meaning of words, bits of words, phrases and sentences
Semantic Pragmatic difficulty/disorder	Children who speak well and clearly but very literally, often saying more than they understand, poor at conversation skills like turn-taking and not knowing when they are not making themselves understood
SENCO	**S**pecial **E**ducational **N**eeds **CO**-ordinator – the member of staff responsible for overseeing special needs provision within a school
Sequencing skills	Ability to place pictures, writing, events, activities or thoughts about any of these in a logical order
Sequential memory	After an activity, event, story, etc. Remembering the main points and re-telling them well
Social use of language SULP/Social Use of Language Programme	Understanding and use of colloquial terms, jokes, jargon and a range of spoken and body language/gesture that reflects language used in social situations
Special Needs/ learning difficulties	Children who have significantly greater difficulty in learning, than most children of the same age
Syntax	The way words and parts of words combine in phrases and sentences
Turn-taking skills	Knowing when it's your turn to speak or join in during a conversation or activity
Vocabulary	Word labels

Other terminology

Attention span	The length of time a child can concentrate on a task
Auditory discrimination	Listening and identifying differences and similarities between sounds
Auditory memory	Hearing, listening, remembering
Auditory perception	Making sense of sounds or spoken language
Auditory recall	Hearing, listening, remembering then telling
Auditory sequencing	Remembering and repeating sounds or words in the right order
Auditory skill	Ability to hear and listen
Behaviour modification	A programme of intervention set up to improve behaviour
Chronological age	Age in years and months at the time of writing
Cognitive development	Thinking and intelligence
Comprehension	Understanding
Concepts	Categories such as 'food' or 'vehicles' Ideas such as 'rough' or 'smooth' Concrete concepts can be seen and touched: Abstract concepts are like 'happiness', 'sadness', 'tired'
Conductive hearing loss	A hearing loss that fluctuates due to Glue Ear or nasal congestion
Co-ordination	Getting different muscles in the body to work together
Cross laterality	Where a child's preferred hand is different from their preferred eye, foot or ear (Right hand/ left foot…)
ENT department	Ear, Nose and Throat department at a hospital
Emotional Behavioural Development (EBD)	How a child feels and behaves. Sometimes EBD is used as shorthand for children with emotional and behavioural difficulties
Fine motor control/function	Ability to control the movement of body (parts) in an accurate manner. Usually, in school, this means hand eye co-ordination in such activities as threading, writing, drawing, cutting, etc.
Gait	The way in which a child walks
Gross motor control/ function/co-ordination	Whole-body movement used for balance, walking, rolling, pedalling a bike, etc.
Global/developmental delay	Children whose overall performance is significantly below that of most children of the same age
Hand dominance	Child's preferred hand in tasks such as cutting, writing, throwing, etc.
IEP	Individual Educational Programme – written outline of a child's own targets
IQ (Intelligent Quotient)	Standardised score from an intelligence test; an average child has an IQ of 100
Laterality	Most people use the same hand/foot/eye for most tasks (either their right or left). Where the dominance is mixed (right hand/left foot, etc.) this is cross laterality, sometimes this causes problems

Mainstream class	A class in an ordinary school, not a specialist unit
Memory skills	Long-term memory – remembering things a long time later Short-term memory – remembering things straight after hearing/seeing them Working memory – Things understood and remembered so they can be used, like using numbers to count rather than just reciting them by rote
Modelling	Showing/demonstrating a task
Motor control	Ability to move whole body/body parts
Ocular motor skills	Co-ordination of hand and eye in tasks such as catching, writing, etc.
One to one	When a child works with the support of one adult – individual support
Overall development/ functioning skills	How a child grows and what is expected at each age in thinking, playing, talking, hearing, seeing, etc.
Overlearning	Giving lots of practice at a task to make sure a child understands it and remembers how to do it
Partial hearing loss	Some but not total hearing loss
Fluctuating hearing loss	Sometimes good hearing, sometimes not. Can be due to "Glue Ear", grommets may be fitted
PHU or HIU	<u>P</u>artial <u>H</u>earing <u>U</u>nit/Hearing Impaired Unit – a small class for children with hearing difficulties
Peers/peer group	Children of the same age
Perceptual skills	Making sense of shapes and patterns in what is seen (visual perception) and what is heard (auditory perception)
Self image/esteem/concept	How a child thinks about him/her self. A child's self-confidence
Siblings	Brothers and sisters
Social skills	Being able to mix with others, knowing how to behave and speak in a range of situations (greetings, joining in games and play, manners and politeness
Symbolic play	Imagining a toy or an object is something else and using it in play – a box to be a car, a leaf to be food, etc.
Tactile skills	Feeling objects to find out about them
Visual acuity	How well a person can see
Visual cues	Pictures, symbols, signs used to prompt memory
Visual defect	Something wrong with eyesight
Visual discrimination	Ability to look for and find differences and similarities in objects, pictures, words, etc.
Visual memory	Remembering how things looked
Visual recall	Remembering and telling how things looked

Books and Resources

2. Expressive Language

Berry, M. (1980) *Teaching Linguistically Handicapped Children* Prentice-Hall

Biddulph, L and McQueen, D. *How to Help Talking* First Community Health, Beecroft Clinic, Cannock Chase Hospital, Brunswick Road, Cannock, Staffordshire WS11 2XY

Catts, H. (1996) 'Defining dyslexia as a developmental language disorder: An expanded view' in *Topics in Language Disorders* 16[2]:14-29

Cooke, J. and Williams, D. (1985) *Working with Children's Language* Winslow Press

Dodd, B. (1994) *Differential Diagnosis and Treatment of Speech Disordered Children* Whurr

Donaldson, M. (1995) *Children with Language Impairment – an introduction* Jessica Kingsley

Hutt, E. (1986) *Teaching Language Disordered Children* Arnold

Law, J. (Ed) (2000) *Communications Difficulties in Childhood* Medical Press

Martin, D and Miller, C. (1996) *Speech and Language Difficulties in the Classroom* David Fulton

Mogford, K and Sadler, J. (1995) *Child Language Disability: Implications in an Educational Setting* Egghead Publications

Moodley, M. and Reynell, J. (1978) *Helping Language Development* Arnold

Pinker, S. (1994) *The Language Instinct* Penguin Books

Snowling, M and Stackhouse, J.(1995) *Dyslexia, Speech and Language: A Practitioner's Book* Whurr

Turnbull, J. and Stewart, T. *Helping Children Cope with Stammering* Sheldon Press

Resources

- **AFASIC**, 2nd floor, 50-52 Great Sutton Street, London. EC1V 0DJ. This is a parent-led organisation that works on behalf of children and young people who have a speech and language difficulty. AFASIC publishes a number of useful leaflets and booklets.
- **Breakthrough to Literacy** available from Longman Group UK Ltd, Longman House, Burnt Mill, Harlow, Essex CM20 2JE
- **Bullying and the Dysfluent Child in the Primary School** The British Stammering Association, 15 Old Ford Road, London E2 9PJ
- **Earwiggo** Lovely Music, 17 Westgate, N. Yorks LS24 9JB A set of six books on rhythm, pitch and simple songs.
- **Early Learning Centre.** The high street shop sells a range of small world toys most useful for language work and we have found their *What Do I Use* game useful too.
- **Functional Language in the Classroom** by Maggie Johnson available from The Department of Psychology and Speech Pathology, The Manchester Metropolitan University, Elizabeth

Gaskell Site, Hathersage Road, Manchester M13 0JA. Ideas and suggestions to improve listening and understanding.

- **Jolly Phonics materials** Jolly Learning Ltd, Tailours House, High Road, Chigwell, Essex IG7 6Dl
- **LDA** Duke Street, Wisbech, Cambs. PE13 2AE or on line at www.instructionalfair.co.uk A wide range of resources to support speech and language work. We have found **Sound Beginnings** – a phonological awareness pack and **LDA Language cards** especially **Social Sequences** and **Actions cards** particularly useful.
- **Living Language & Teaching Talking** by Ann Locke, NFER Nelson, 2 Oxford Road East, Windsor, Berkshire SL4 1DF or online at edu&hsc@nfer-nelson.co.uk
- **Orchard Toys**, Formlend Ltd, Keyworth, Nottingham but also available from high street shops. We have found their **Quack Quack** and **Insy Winsy games** very useful.
- **Order Order** – photocopiable sequencing sheets available from Easy Learn, Trent House, Fiskerton, Southwell, Nottinghamshire NG25 0UH
- **PORIC** by Glinette Woods & Deborah Acors – **Language Concepts** In addition photocopiable **Language Concepts Books 1-4** and **Past Tense and Concept** Calendar Nutshell Services, Blake End, Essex CM7 8SH
- **The Language Gap** available from SENTER Freepost NT 2550, Whitley Bay NE26 1BR. Photocopiable games and pictures for Language development (auditory memory, verbal reasoning, sequencing)
- Ravensburger games are available from high street shops we have found **What's my name** and **Tell a story** very useful.
- **Sequencing stories** – Photocopiable sequencing material at three levels available from Learning Materials Ltd, Dixon Street, Wolverhampton WV2 2BX
online at Learning.Materials@btinternet.com
- **Song books** to support language development both from A & C Black, 33 Bedford Row, London, WC1R 4JH: *Bingo Lingo* by Helen MacGregor ISBN:0-7136-5075-3 *Michael Finnigin, Tap your Chinigin* by Sue Nicholls ISBN 0 7136 4716 7
- **Speechmark Publishing** – A range of books and products Telford Road, Bicester, Oxon OX26 4LQ or online at www.speechmark.net
- **STASS**, 44 North Road, Ponteland, Northumberland NE20 9UR A range of resources to support speech and language work. We have found **Semantic Links** and the **Teddy Language Pack** particularly useful.
- **Winslow** Press, Goytside Road, Chesterfield, Derbyshire S40 2PH A wide range of resources to support speech and language work.

Amendment to page 122

PORIC by Glinette Woods and Deborah Acors – **Concepts instruction book** (plus cross-referenced photocopiable **Concept Consolidation Books 1–4, Past Tense Consolidation and Concept Calendar**) Cheerful Publications, 7 Oxley Close, Gidea Park, Romford, Essex RM2 6NX

3. Receptive Language

Books and Resources

Many of the books and resources for Expressive Language given above contain information and ideas for Receptive Language development.

In addition

- **Paget Gorman Signed Speech** – Paget Gorman Society, 2 Dowlands Bungalows, Dowlands Lane, Smallfields RH6 9SD
  Cued Articulation, Jane Passey, Stass publications, 44 North Road, Ponteland Northumberland NE20 9UR
- **Functional Language in the Classroom** by Maggie Johnson available from Janine Acott, The Department of Psychology and Speech Pathology, The Manchester Metropolitan University, Elizabeth Gaskell Site, Hathersage Road, Manchester M13 0JA
- **Glue Ear – Guidelines for teachers**. Leaflet available from The Hearing Research Trust, 330-332 Gray's Inn Road, London WC1X 8EE
- **Leap into Listening** – photocopiable listening activities from **Winslow (See above)**
- **Listen and Do** from LDA (See above)
- **Listening Skills Early Years** and **Listening Skills Key Stage 1** – Photocopiable sheets for listening activities/tasks. Available from Questions Publishing Company, Leonard House, 321, Bradford St, Birmingham B5 6ET www.education-quest.com
- **Reading for Meaning, Sound Lotto etc.** from Learning Materials Ltd, Dixon Street, Wolverhampton WV2 2BX or on line at learning.materials@btinternet.com
- **What am I?** – listening game with cassette and cards from Early Learning Centre shops

4. Social Use of Language Skills

Books

Anderson-Wood, L. and Rae Smith, B. *Working with Pragmatics* Winslow Press

Bliss,T. and Tetley, J. *Circle Time* and *Developing Circle Time* Lucky Duck Publishing

Conti-Ramsden, G. and McTear, M. (1992) *Pragmatic disorders in Children – Assessment and Intervention* Whurr

Firth, C. and Venkatesh, K. *Semantic-Pragmatic Language Disorder Resource Pack* Winslow Press

Frances, J. and Brownsword, K. *A Positive Approach* Belair

Goodwin J. *100 Games* Headstart, East London

Gray, C. *The New Social Story Book* Winslow Press

Grundy, P. *Doing Pragmatics* Arnold

Lucas, E. *Semantic Pragmatic Language Disorders* Aspen, USA

Martin, D and Miller, C. *Speech and Language Difficulties in the Classroom* David Fulton

Mildred, M. *Let's Play Together* Green Print

Mortimer, H. *Learning Through Play – Circle Time* Scholastic

Moseley, J. *Quality Circle Time, More Quality Circle Time* LDA

Oldham Speech Therapy Department. *Hold my glasses and don't nibble the ends* A practical guide to working with semantic pragmatic language disordered children. Speech Therapy Dept. Oldham N.H.S. Trust, Oldham.

Rowe, C. 'Do Social Stories Benefit Children with Autism in Mainstream Schools' in *British Journal of Special Education* March 1999

Rustin, L. and Kuhr, A. *Social Skills and the Speech Impaired* Whurr

Sher, B. *Popular Games for Positive Play Therapy* Skill Builders (Psychological Corporation) and *Self Esteem Games* John Wiley & Sons

Resources

- **Celebrations** – A book of photocopiable certificates by George Robinson and Barbara Maines from Lucky Duck Publications, 10 South Terrace, Redland, Bristol BS6 6TG
- **Mad, Sad, Glad** game, Emotions photo cards from Winslow Press
- **Praise Postcards,** The Primary Print People, 142 Blackburn road, Bolton, Lancashire BL1 8DR
- **RoSPA** catalogue with a range of useful resources available from RoSPA, Edgbaston Park, 353 Bristol Road, Birmingham B5 7ST or online at www.rospa.co.uk
- **Superstickers,** PO Box 55, 4 Balloo Avenue, Bangor, County Down BT19 7PJ as they have a "I listen carefully" badge.
- **The Giggly, Grumpy, Scary Book** – A songbook with CD Universal Edition, London
- **A teacher made toolkit for circle games** is useful, mine includes:
  blindfold
  set of keys
  large foam ball
  magic wand
  soft toy/shell or similar to pass round when talking round the circle
  clear photos/pictures of happy/sad etc.
  favourite book, toy, colour, food etc.

5. Developmental Co-ordination Difficulties

Books

Beattie, L. *Tips with Teens* Dyspraxia Foundation

Dennison, P. and Dennison, G. *Brain Gym* Body Balance Books, 12 Golders Rise, London NW4 2HR

Kirby, A. *Dyspraxia – The Hidden handicap* Human Horizon Series

Kranowitz, C. *The Out of Sync Child* Berkley Publishing Group

Marshall, L. *Handwriting Activities* from Communications Manager, Education Dept, The Castle, Winchester, Hampshire SO23 8UG

Macintyre, C. *Dyspraxia in the Early Years* David Fulton

Meister-Vitale, B. *Unicorns are real – A Right Brained Approach to Learning* Falmer Press

Oakes Park School and Support Service. *Working with Clumsy Children, A Practical approach for Teachers* Available from Oakes Park School and Support Service, Matthews Lane, Sheffield S88JJ

Poustie, J. *Life Skills – Practical Solutions for Specific Learning Difficulties* Dyspraxia Foundation

Ripley, K Daines, B, Barett, J.*Inclusion for Children with Dyspraxia / DCD A Handbook for Teachers* David Fulton

Russell, J.P. (1988) *Graded activities for Children with Motor Difficulties* Cambridge University Press

SENSS North Lincolnshire *Supporting the child with dyspraxia in the mainstream classroom* SENSS, Educational Development Centre, South Leys Campus, Enderby Road, Scunthorpe, N Lincolnshire DN17 2JL

Witherick, S. *Assessment and Activities for Hand Skills and Fine Motor development – A practical guide for teachers* ReLeass c/o Educational Services, 10-12 George Hudson Street, York YO1 6ZG

Resources

- **Anything Left Handed** 18, Avenue Road, Belmont Surrey, SM2 6JD A range of resources for left-handers.
- **Dextral books** (Incorporating The Left Handed Company) PO Box 52, South Do, Manchester, M20 2PJ A range of resources for left-handers including sloping boards that I adapt for right handers.
- **The Dyspraxia Foundation** is a national charity that supports and informs those concerned with Dyspraxia (DCD). It publishes a number of useful leaflets, booklets and books.
- **Easylearn**, Trent House, Fiskerton, Southwell, Nottinghamshire, NG25 0UH or online at enquiry@easylearn.co.uk. A range of useful photocopiable resources including **Fine Motoring** – photocopiable sheets with a range of fine motor skills.
- Gymnic/Epsan Waterfly UK Ltd Anglo House, Worcester Road, Stourport on Severn DY13 9AW or online at salesuk@epsan waterfly.com. **Movin'sit posture cushions** and many more resources to support the development of co-ordination and movement skills.
- **LDA** A range of useful products including: **Let's Look**, Photocopiable visual discrimination sheets.
  Lined paper – helpful guidelines for writing.
  Write from the Start [formerly Theoderescu] – photocopiable booklets to help develop fine motor and perceptual skills.
  Tri-go grip – the pencil grip we have found to be most effective with right or left-handers.
- **Rompa Ltd** Goytside Road, Chesterfield, Derbyshire S40 2PH Resources to support the development of co-ordination and movement skills.
- **Resources for Schools,** Folk in Education 4, Mill Lane, Much Cowarne near Bromyard, Herefordshire HR7 4JH Music and dance resources including **Fun Folk Dances** by Marion Percy – Twelve very simple folk dances, some based on nursery rhymes, good for rhythm and for direction, sequencing and learning left and right.
- **Taskmaster Ltd,** Morris Road, Leicester LE2 6BR
- **The Happy Puzzle Company** Mail order from The Happy Puzzle Company Ltd, PO Box 24041 London NW4 2ZN or online at www.happypuzzle.co.uk Puzzles and games some of which are useful for developing manipulative and motor planning skills.

6. Curriculum

English
Books

Barrs, M. and Thomas, A. *The Reading Book* Centre for Language in Primary Education, Webber Row, London SE1 8QW

Goswami, U. and Bryant, P. *Phonological Skills and Learning to Read* ErIbaum, New York

Layton, L. Deeny, K. and Upton, G. *Sound Practice. Phonological Awareness in the Classroom* David Fulton

Lloyd, P. Mitchell, H. and Monk, J. *The Literacy Hour and Language Knowledge* David Fulton

Reason, R. & Boote, R. *Helping Children with Reading and Spelling – A Special Needs Manual* Routledge

Snowling, M. J. *Children's Written Language Difficulties* NFER Nelson

Resources

- **A Helping Hand for Teachers** – A phonic spelling programme from SENTER. Freepost NT 2550, Whitley Bay NE26 1BR
- **Breakthrough to Literacy** available from Longman Group UK Ltd, Longman House, Burnt Mill, Harlow, Essex CM20 2JE
- **Children's Cassettes**/Cover to Cover Cassettes Ltd, PO Box 112, Marlborough, Wiltshire SN8 3UG The Audio Book Collection, FREEPOST (BA1686/1) Bath BA1 3QZ
- **Clicker 4**. Crick Software Ltd. www.cricksoft.com or 35 Charter Gate, Quarry Park Close, Moulton Park, Northampton NN3 6QB
- **Cloze Encounters and Write Now** – Graded cloze exercises and pictures & key words. Precise Educational, Willowbank House Golden Valley, Alfreton, Derbyshire DE55 4ES9
- **Gamz** – Swap and fix spelling/phonic card games that the children can play with minimum supervision. Also games on CD Rom. Gamz, 25 Albert Park Road, Malvern, Worcestershire WR14 1HW
- **Book Bands for Guided Reading** – Grading books to match the needs of the reader in KS1. The Reading Recovery National Network: Institute of Education's Bookshop Tel: 0171 612 6050
- **The NASEN A-Z**: A graded list of reading books from NASEN House, 4-5 Amber Business Village, Amber Close, Amington, Tamworth, Staffs B77 4RP
- **The Core Book List** edited by Ellis and Barrs from The Centre for Language in Primary Education, Webber Street, London SE1 8QW
- **Let's Look** – photocopiable masters for visual discrimination activities LDA
- **Let's Spell** – 5 books (3 letter words, Words that start with a blend, Words that end with a blend, Words that start and end with a blend, words with double vowels). From Smart Kids UK Ltd, 169B Main Street, New Greenham Park, Thatcham, Berkshire RG19 6HN or on line at www.smartkidscatalog.com
- **Language Through Drawing & Language Through Reading** available through ICAN, 4 Dyers Buildings, Holborn, London EC1N 2QP
- **Phonic Activities 1 & 2**. Brighter Vision ISBN: 1-8617-2023-8
- **Photocopiable spelling / phonic books** from letter sounds through

to silent letters from Easy Learn, Trent House, Fiskerton, Southwell, Nottinghamshire NG25 0UH
- **Sound Beginnings** LDA
- **Spelling systems**
  Alpha to Omega Hornsby, B.
  Toe by Toe, Cowling, K. 8 Green Road, Baildon, Shipley, West Yorks BD17 5HL
- **Integrated Learning System.** Systems Integrated Research, 4th Floor, East Mill, Bridgefoot, Belper, Derbyshire DE56 1XQ
- **The First 100 Words** – Core vocabulary, photocopiable, from SENTER. Freepost NT 2550, Whitley Bay NE26 1BR
- **The Whiz Kids** – A series of attractive photocopiable books containing story-based exercises including tracking, classification, following instructions, prediction, cloze and deduction. Learning Materials Ltd, Dixon Street, Wolverhampton WV2 2BX or on line at learning.materials@btinternet.com
- **Timesavers Phonics Books 1-6** and **Write about the picture** – photocopiable masters, Precise Educational, Willowbank House, 19 Golden Valley, Riddings, Derbyshire DE55 4ES
- **Story frames** from Easy Learn, Trent House, Fiskerton, Southwell, Nottinghamshire NG25 0UH
- **Writing Frames for Infants** – photocopiable and CD Rom from Belair Publications, Albert House, Apex Business Centre, Boscombe Road, Dunstable, Beds LU5 4RL or on line at belair-publications.co.uk
- And I have picked up some real bargains in Pound Shops!
  I Can Learn – rhyming cards
  Beginning to Read – Silent "e" card pack

Mathematics
Books

Atkinson, S. (Ed.) *Mathematics and Reason* Hodder and Stoughton
Cook, G. Jones, L. Murphy, C. and Thumpston, G. *Enriching Early Mathematical Learning* OUP
Grauberg, E. (1998) *Elementary Maths and Language Difficulties* Whurr.
El-Naggar, O. (1996) *Specific Learning Difficulties in Mathematics: A Classroom Approach* NASEN
MacGregor, H. *Tom Thumb's Musical Maths* A & C Black

Resources

- **A-Z of maths games** by Karen Breitbart, a selection of simple maths games published by Brilliant Publications, The Old School Yard, Leighton Road, Northall, Dunstable, Bedfordshire LU6 2HA
- **BBC Video Plus Numbertime,** BBC Educational Information, BBC White City, London W12 7TS
- **Maths schemes** – At Key Stage 1 we have found Scottish Primary Maths and Heinemann Maths particularly useful: Heinemann, Halley Court, Jordan Hill, Oxford OX2 8EJ Also Easylearn Maths, Number Books: 1-3 Trent House, Fiskerton, Southwell, Nottinghamshire NG25 0UH and Ginn's Abacus scheme, particularly their Simmering book of short, oral maths activities.

Ginn, Linacre House, Jordan Hill, Oxford OX2 8DP

- **Maths Now – a maths series for Key Stage 2 & 3** written with special needs/language difficulties in mind. John Murray Publishers Ltd, 50 Albemarle Street, London W1X 4BD
- **Talking Maths pictures** from LDA

There is a wide range of maths resources available from a number of companies and some can be easily made. We have found the following particularly useful:

- A range of counters – buttons, bottle tops, sticks…
- A range of teacher-made number lines and number squares
- Sandpaper numerals – available from Philip & Tacey Ltd, North Way, Andover, Hants SP10 5BA
- Number stamps – we purchased some excellent ones from Kershaws Rubber Stamps, Plane Tree, Goose House Lane, Darwen BB3 0EH
- Sumthings – excellent counters, which are on a string rather like rosary beads, so can be moved up and down the string yet hold their position. Available from St Joseph's Workshops, 90 Bagg Lane, Atherton, Manchester
- Multilink cubes, unifix or similar with 1-10 trays
- Cuisenaire rods
- Logiblocks
- Dominoes
- Large dice
- Beads for threading and pattern cards
- A set of measuring containers plus everyday containers that the children are familiar with – shampoo bottles, pop bottles etc.
- Balance scales, weights and a selection of items to weigh including teacher-made parcels. We have two types of parcel – a set of small, same-sized boxes with different items put inside, making them different weights, and a set of different sized parcels where some big parcels are very light and some small parcels are very heavy
- Individual clocks with analog and digital. These can be simply made by buying or photocopying and laminating analog clocks, then adding a strip of white card at the bottom with two central dots. This can then be used as a whiteboard digital clock
- 1 minute and 5 minute timers, a kitchen timer and a stop clock
- Commercial solid shapes and a set of environmental solid shapes, things the children will be familiar with – cylindrical felt pens, coins/cuboid books, boxes/cube oxo cubes, bricks… to help them make connections between their maths shape vocabulary and their world
- Plastic coins and real coins

Science
Books and Resources

- **Naturetrek Science Resource books** – Key Stages 1 & 2. These are excellent for teaching, recording and assessment. Naturetrek Educational, St Asaph, Denbighshire, North Wales LL17 0AZ
- **Science for Children with Learning Difficulties** Simon & Schuster
- **Science Sequencing Pictures** – very useful picture sequences of seed to plant, caterpillar to butterfly etc though this is an American publication so you need to change some vocabulary e.g. Fall to Autumn. and **The Big Book of Science Rhymes and Chants** by Jo Ellen Moore & Leslie Tryon. Available through Scholastic Publications, Villiers House, Clarendon Avenue, Leamington Spa, Warwickshire CV32 5PR
- **Scholastic Publications** also produce a range of useful books:
  Seeds and Seedlings
  Pushing and Pulling
  Light and Colour
- **Science videos** – The BBC produce a number of very useful:
  Materials & their uses
  Electricity, Light & Sound
  People & Living
  Forces & Weather
  BBC Video Plus, BBC Educational Information, BBC White City, London W12 7TS

There is a wide range of science resources available from a number of companies and we have access to our mainstream school stock of these but in addition we wouldn't be without:

- A set of toys collected from charity shops and school fairs that are used during work on Forces and Motion and Electricity
- A set of lights old and new and reflective toys/ornaments – candles, torches, kaleidoscopes, different mirrors, … that are used during work on Light
- A class percussion and music-making set that are used during work on Sound
- A set of items made from different materials both manmade and natural that is used during work on Materials
- A class gardening kit that is used during work on Life and Living Things

All of the above are used for vocabulary work and in addition we have sets of items for particular vocabulary/concepts:

- Rough/smooth
- Hard/soft
- Wet/dry

These are ready prepared for teaching and as 'hands on' displays.

- **Guess Who** – Hasbro UK Ltd, Caswell way, Newport, Gwent NP9 0YH also available from the Early Learning Centre
- **History/Geography videos** – The BBC produce a number of very useful titles:
  90 years ago with Magic Grandad
  Seaside holidays with Magic Grandad
  Within living memory
  Famous events
  Famous people
  BBC Video Plus, BBC Educational Information, BBC White City, London W12 7TS
- **Legend into Language** – Myths & Legends at Key Stages 1 & 2 Belair Publications Ltd ISBN 0 947882 69 3
- **Long ago and far away** – activities using stories for History & Geography at Key Stage 1 Developmental Educational Centre, Gillett Centre, 998 Bristol Road, Selly Oak,Birmingham B29 6LE
- **Musical starting Points with Young Children** Ward Locke
- **Sense of History Series** at Key Stages 1 & 2, Longman School's Division, Harlow, Essex CM20 2YF
- **Starting with me** – Topic ideas for History, Geography & RE at Key Stage 1 Belair Publications Ltd ISBN 0 947882 18 9
- **Talking History pictures** from LDA
- **The Excellence of Play** by Janet Moyle (1993) OUP
- **Three Singing Pigs** by Kaye Umansky – Music & Traditional Stories A & C Black, London ISBN 0 7136 3804 4
- **Small Steps Forward** by Sarah Newman (1999) Jessica Kingsley

7. Parents as Part of the Team

- Blamires, M. Robertson, C, Blamires, J. (1997) *Parent Teacher Partnership* David Fulton
- Gascoigne, E. (1995) *Working with Parents as Partners* in SEN David Fulton Publishing

Useful addresses

AFASIC Association For All Speech Impaired Children, 2nd floor, 50-52 Great Sutton Street, London EC1V 0DJ
Much useful information and legal support about speech and language impairment, magazine produced and conferences held.

Contact a Family 170 Tottenham Court Road, London W1P 0HA
Co-ordinates a network of 800 local support groups for parents of children with special needs.

British Dyslexia Association (BDA) 98 London Road, Reading, Berkshire RG1 5AU

Dyslexia Institute 133 Gresham Road, Staines, Middlesex TW18 2AJ

Dyspraxia Foundation 8 West Alley, Hitchin, Hertfordshire SG5 1EG
Much useful information about Developmental Co-ordination Difficulties, magazine produced and conferences held.

ICAN – Invalid Children's Aid Nationwide. 4 Dyer's Building, Holborn London EC1N 2QP
Much useful information about Speech and Language Impairment, magazine produced and training sessions held.

NAPLIC – National Association of Professionals concerned with Language Impaired Children. c/o Glinette Woods, 32 Arlington Gardens, Harold Wood, Romford RM3 0EA
NAPLIC issue a bulletin three times a year and hold an annual conference and their post conference papers are most useful.

NASEN (National Association for Special Educational Needs). NASEN House, 4/5 Amber Business Village, Amington, Tamworth, Staffs B77 4RP
Information about special educational needs, magazine produced and conferences held.

National Autistic Society 276 Willesden Lane, London NW2 5RB
A range of useful information, including a paper on the overlaps between Autism and Speech and Language Impairment.

National Listening Library 12 Lane Street, London SE1
It is possible, for £25 a year, to borrow a tape machine and story tapes so that a child may read andlisten at the same time. An application must be supported by a teacher, doctor or otherprofessional.

Parents in Partnership Unit 2, Ground Floor, 70 South Lambeth Road, London SW8 1RL
Parents' support organisation which offers information and support.

Questions Publishing Leonard House, 321 Bradford Street, Digbeth, Birmingham B5 6ET or online at www.education-quest.com
Monthly magazine – *Special Children*, other educational magazines and resources.

SNIP – Special Needs Information Press Spring Cottage, Bagot Street, Abbots Bromley, Staffordshire WS15 3DA
A newsletter for all those working with pupils with special needs, packed with information for a reasonable subscription.

The Turner Library Whitefields Schools and Centre, MacDonald Road, Walthamstow, London E17 4AZ
If you would like to keep up to date with the latest research in special

needs, including Speech and Language, for a reasonable membership fee and between 20p and £1 per page, this library can provide copies of articles from a range of journals. A bulletin is issued bimonthly.

Write Away 29 Crawford Street, London W1H 1PL The penfriend scheme for adults and children with disabilities or special needs

Useful websites

AFASIC – promotes understanding, awareness of speech and language impairment and equal opportunities for those with speech and language impairment www.afasic.org.uk

Badger books – Books on sensitive issues. www.badger-publishing.co.uk

BBC Online Education – www.bbc.co.uk/education/

BECTA Special Needs and Inclusion – a range of information about using ICT to support learners with special needs. www.becta.org.uk/inclusion/

British Dyslexia Association (BDA) – www.bda-dyslexia.org.uk

Centre for Studies on Inclusive Education (CSIE) – inclusion.uwe.ac.uk

Code of Practice – dfee.gov.uk/sen

Communication Matters – information about Augmentative and Alternative Communication www.communicationmatters.org.uk

Contact a Family – support and advice for parents of children with special needs www.cafamily.org.uk

Crick Software – free downloadable resources on their Clicker Grids for Learning www.cricksoft.com

David Fulton Publishers – specialise in special education books www.fultonbooks.co.uk

Dyslexia.com – www.dyslexic.com

Dyspraxia Foundation – www.emmbrook.demon.co.uk/dysprax/homepage.htm

Granada Learning/SEMERC – ICT and special needs. www.granadalearning.com/special_needs

National Association for Special Educational Needs (NASEN) www.nasen.org.uk

National Autistic Society – www.oneworld.org/autism.uk

Oaasis (Office for Advice Assistance Support and Information) www.oaasis.co.uk

Picture Exchange System (PECS) – information about specialised use of pictures/symbols with children with communication difficulties. www.pecs-uk.com

PIPPY – American site with lots of ideas. www.aacintervention.com

Questions Publishing Online – www.education-quest.com

Special Education Exchange – www.spedex.com

Special Needs Directory – www.canterbury.ac.uk/xplanatory/xplan.htm

Anything Left Handed 18 Avenue Road, Belmont, Surrey SM2 6JD A wide range of resources for left-handers.

Belair Publications Albert House, Apex Business Centre, Boscombe Road, Dunstable, Beds. LU5 4RL or on line at www.belair-publications.co.uk A range of curriculum information/ideas books, particularly useful for art/design and displays.

Dextral Books (incorporating The Left Handed Company) Dextral Books, PO Box 52, South Do, Manchester M20 2PJ Books, Handwriting resources, Left Handed resources.

Early Learning Centre on your high street or on line at www.elc.co.uk A range of games useful for vocabulary and turntaking.

Easylearn Easy Learn, Trent House, Fiskerton, Southwell, Nottinghamshire NG25 0UH or on line at www.easylearn.co.uk A range of photocopiable special educational needs materials at reasonable prices.

David Fulton Publishers Ltd Ormond House, 26-27 Boswell Street, London WC1N 3JZ or on line atwww.fultonpublishers.co.uk A comprehensive selection of books on special educational needs including speech and language impairment, it's well worthwhile obtaining a catalogue.

Gamz 25 Albert Park Road, Malvern, Worcestershire WR14 1HW A range of easy to play/self-checking spelling/phonic card games.

Hands On Unit 11 Tannery Road, Tonbridge, Kent, TN9 1RF A range of educational resources.

LDA Duke Street, Wisbech, Cambs. PE13 2AE or on line at www.instructionalfair.co.uk. A range of special educational needs materials.

Learning Materials Ltd Dixon Street, Wolverhampton WV2 2BX A range of special educational needs materials at reasonable prices.

Precise Educational Willowbank House Golden Valley, Alfreton, Derbyshire DE55 4ES A range of photocopiable special educational needs materials.

Questions Publishing Leonard House, 321 Bradford Street, Digbeth, Birmingham B5 6ET

Rompa Goyt Side Road, Chesterfield, Derbyshire S40 2PH or online at www.rompa.com Products, services for people with special needs, sensory impairment and learning disabilities.

S&S Services Station Road, Harvington, Evesham, Worcestershire WR11 5NJ or on line at www.ss-services.co.uk A range of craft resources, including reasonably priced calendars.

SEN Marketing 618 Leeds Road, Outwood, Wakefield WF1 2LT or online at www.sen.uk.com Dyslexia and Special Needs Bookshop.

SENTER Freepost NT 2550, Whitley Bay NE26 1BR A range of photocopiable resources for special needs.

Smartkids 169b Main Street, New Greenham Park, Thatcham, Berkshire RG19 6HN or on line at www.smartkidscatalog.com A range of special educational needs materials.

Speechmark Publishing – A range of books and products Telford Road, Bicester, Oxon OX26 4LQ or online at www.speechmark.net

STASS 44 North Road, Ponteland, Northumberland NE20 9UR A range of resources to support speech and language work, including Paget Gorman materials. We have found Semantic Links and the Teddy Language Pack particularly useful.

Taskmaster Ltd Morris Road, Leicester LE2 6BR or online at www.besanet.org.uk A range of special educational needs materials with a section on speech/auditory skills.

Winslow Goytside Road, Chesterfield, Derbyshire S40 2PH A range of special educational needs resources for sensory motor, speech and language, social and emotional and much more.

Further reading

The ones in green are particularly suitable for parents.

Bell, F. *Red Pages – A Guide to Children's Books Relevant to Special Needs* from Bradhill Books, Chipping Norton

Beveridge, M. and Conti-Ramsden, G. (1986) *Children with Language Disabilities* Arnold, Open University

Bloom, L. and Lahey, M. (1978) *Language Development and Language Disorders* Wiley

Browning, E. (1987) *I Can't See What You're Saying* Angel Press/Hotten Street Press, Slough

Byers-Brown, B. and Edwards, M. (1989) *Developmental Disorders of Language* Whurr

Capelin, S. *Rachel: the write to speak* from Sandra Capelin, Mount Pleasant, Darite, Liskeard, Cornwall PL14 5JW

Cline, T. and Baldwin, S. (1994) *Selective Mutism in Children* Whurr

Crystal, D. (1987) *Child Language Learning and Linguistics* Arnold

Crystal, D. (1986) *Listen to Your Child – A Parent's Guide to Children's Language* Penguin

Cumine, V. Leach, J. and Stevenson, G. (1998) *Asperger Syndrome – A Practical Guide for Teachers* David Fulton

Cunningham, C. and Davis, H. (1985) *Working with Parents* Open University Press

Donaldson, M (1986) *Children's Minds.* Glasgow: Collins/Fontana

Fletcher, P. and Hall, D. (1992) *Specific Speech and Language Disorders in Children* Whurr

Hughes, Althea. (1982) *I Can't Talk Like You* Suitable to be read to children. Dinosaur Publications.

Jeffree, D. and McConkey, R. *Let Me Speak* Human Horizons

Kersner, M. and Wright, J. (Editors). (1993) *How to Manage Communication Problems in Young Children* Winslow

Law James, Parkinson Alison with Tamhne Rashmin (Editors) (2000) *Communication Difficulties in Childhood – A Practical Guide* Radcliffe Medical Press

Lebrun, Y. (1990) *Mutism.* Whurr

Lees, J. and Urwin, S. (1991) *Children with Language Disorders* Whurr

McAleer Hamaguchi, P. (1995) *Childhood Speech, Language and Listening Problems* Wiley and Sons, New York

Mogford, K. and Sadler, J. (1989) *Child Language Disability* Multilingual Matters

Yule, W. and Rutter, M. (1987) *Language Development and Disorder.* MacKeith Press, London

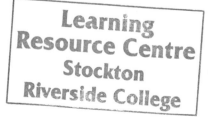

Structured Activities for Language and Literacy in the Early Years

"Children make significant gains in phonological awareness"

A complete package to prepare nursery-aged children for the demands of the literacy hour. The **SALLEY** programme can be used by any early years practitioner. It is both a prevention and intervention programme designed to teach the phonological awareness skills that are so fundamental to the development of reading and spelling.

It has been widely trialled in nursery and reception classes.

Handbook: explaining the background to the original research.

Cassette: a recording of everyday sounds.

Manual: detailing the content of each daily session and instructions for delivery.

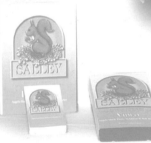

Video: showing examples of the programme tasks.

Puppet: SALLEY squirrel is a lovable, furry glove puppet.

Order form

I wish to order _____ SALLEY toolkits at £95.00 plus VAT (Total £105.00) per set, plus £5.00 p&p (£7.00 overseas)

Name: _____

Job Title: _____

Delivery address: _____

_____

_____ Postcode: _____

Tel no: _____

Email: _____

Completed forms may be posted to:
The Questions Publishing Company Ltd, Leonard House, 321 Bradford Street, Digbeth, Birmingham B5 6ET

Credit card hotline: 0121 666 7878
Fax orders: 0121 666 7879

I enclose a cheque made payable to Questions Publishing Company Ltd the sum of £ _____

☐ I enclose an official order No. _____

☐ I wish to pay by Mastercard ☐ Visa ☐ Switch ☐

Credit card No:

☐☐☐☐☐☐☐☐☐☐☐☐☐☐☐☐☐☐☐

Expiry date: ☐☐☐☐   Issue No: ☐☐

Signature: _____

If paying by credit card, please give name and address if different from delivery address.

Name on card: _____

Address: _____

_____ Postcode: _____

Tel no: _____   Email: _____

Special CHILDREN

Supporting Children Series

The *Supporting Children* books are aimed at educational practitioners, both teachers and learning assistants, in specialist and non-specialist settings. Each book provides theory to inform the reader about a specific special need, while the main body of the text offers practical advice, support and activities to facilitate pupils' learning.

Coming soon:

Supporting Children with Dyslexia

Supporting Children with ADHD

This book, with an introduction for teachers, is a photocopiable resource for children with ADHD. The activities and advice aim to enable these children to control their own feelings, thoughts and actions. By working through the activities, pupils will improve their self-esteem and understand their personality type.

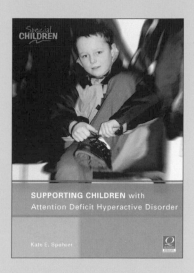

Price: £14.99 **ISBN:** 1-84190-056-7 **Format:** A4 Approx. 88pp

Supporting Children with Autism in Mainstream Schools

It is increasingly common for children with autism to attend mainstream schools. Using the child-centred, whole-school approach provided in this resource, teachers will be able to implement strategies for supporting these children in the classroom, and successfully meeting their learning needs.

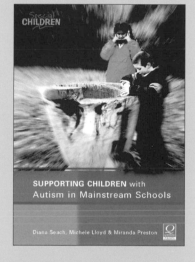

Price: £14.99 **ISBN:** 1-84190-055-9 **Format:** A4 Approx. 80pp

Supporting Children with Multiple Disabilities

By following the practical framework provided, teachers will be able to implement a multi-sensory curriculum in the classroom. This will enable children with multiple disabilities to become more independent and active, and to develop effective communication skills.

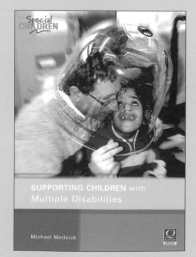

Price: £14.99 **ISBN:** 1-84190-042-7 **Format:** A4 Approx. 180pp

Order form

I wish to place an order for the following titles:

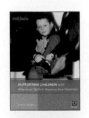 Supporting Children with ADHD   copies
£14.99

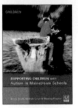 Supporting Children with Autism   copies
in Mainstream Schools
£14.99

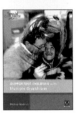 Supporting Children with   copies
Multiple Difficulties
£14.99

PLEASE SEND MY ORDER TO:

Name: _____

Job title: _____

Delivery address: _____

_____

Postcode: _____

Tel: _____   Fax: _____

Email: _____

For Postage & Packing please add £3.00 U.K. £5.00 Overseas

☐ I enclose a cheque for £_____

made payable to The Questions Publishing Company Ltd.

☐ I wish to pay by credit card:

No. ☐☐☐☐☐☐☐☐☐☐☐☐☐☐☐☐☐☐☐

Expiry date: ☐☐☐☐   Signature: _____

Please give card address if different from delivery address:

_____

_____

Postcode: _____   Tel: _____

☐ I wish to pay by Official Order no. _____

**Credit Card Hotline
0121 666 7878**

Fax orders 0121 666 7879

Email sales@questpub.co.uk

Return completed form to
The Questions Publishing Company Ltd,
1st Floor, Leonard House,
321 Bradford Street,
Digbeth, Birmingham B5 6ET